Rare Threads:
A Life with Prader-Willi Syndrome

Sebastiaan van Nuissenburg

Copyright © 2024 (Sebastiaan van Nuissenburg)
All rights reserved worldwide.

No part of this publication may be reproduced, stored in a retrieval system, or transmitted, in any form or by any means, electronic, mechanical, photocopying, recording or otherwise, without the express written permission of the author. No use of artificial intelligence (ai) in writing of this book.

Edited by
Kaaren Sutcliffe at Just So Words

Prepublication Data Service
P.O. Box 159, Calwell, ACT Australia 2905
Email: publishaspg@gmail.com
http://www.inspiringpublishers.com

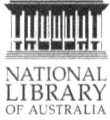 A catalogue record for this book is available from the National Library of Australia

National Library of Australia The Prepublication Data Service

Author: Sebastiaan van Nuissenburg
Title: Rare Threads: A Life with Prader-Willi Syndrome
Genre: Nonfiction

Paperback ISBN: 978-1-923087-17-0
PDF eBook ISBN: 978-1-923087-16-3
ePub2 ISBN: 978-1-923087-15-6

Contents

Dedication……………………………………………………………………v
Foreword……………………………………………………………………vii
Disclaimer methods………………………………………………………ix
About the Author…………………………………………………………xi
Indomitable Caregivers …………………………………………………xii

The phone call at 14:35……………………………………………………1
A World of Challenges and Uncertain Magic………………………13
Taking on the Journey……………………………………………………19
Early Years and Growing Challenges – Age One …………………27
Coping Strategies and Adjustments – Age Two……………………33
The Awakening - Age Three ……………………………………………43
The Dark Waters of Hunger - Age Four ……………………………51
Breaking the Cycle - Age Four…………………………………………56
The Discovery - Age Five ………………………………………………63
The Mystoria School of Magic - Day One - Age Six ………………71
The Department of Paediatric Wizardry,
and the Department of Linguistic Charms - Age Six ……………77
The Struggles of Structure and Communication -
Age Seven……………………………………………………………………85
The Call to Adventure - Age Seven……………………………………91
The Quest for the Magical Guardian -
Defence Against the Dark Arts position……………………………97

Unraveling the Mystery - Age Eight 105
The Spell of Change - Age Nine 111
A Scholarly Odyssey - Age Ten 117
Mission. Values. Vision. 127
BUD/RATs™ Training 131
Feeling Good, Looking Good, Oughta be in Hollywood 135
Understanding Behavioural Problems & the Six Levels
of Disquietude.. 155
Techniques for Parents... 161
The Sequential Positive Behaviour Management Program........ 165
The five steps 168
More useful tips 178
The Morning Tasks.. 181
The Afternoon Tasks 183
When Challenges Overwhelm Facing the Hard Truths
of Maturity 187
Exploring Emotional Regulation with GABA and Concerta........ 191
A Hundred Days of Transformation:
Aston-Martin's Journey with GABA 194
Proposing an Advanced Diploma in Behavioural
Therapy with a Genetic and Chromosomal Emphasis 199
You're my one in 8 billion - My closing moments 205

Dedication

My dearest son, Aston-Martin,

This book, a labour of love, has been a decade in the making. Yet, it is you who has given me the most incredible ten years a father could ever hope for, and I eagerly anticipate the many more still to come. I have never once given up on you, and I never will. Your radiant smile each morning, the sound of your laughter when you reunite with daddy, the joy you bring to others by being their friend and making them smile, and the warmth of your hugs and our playful tag games – these cherished moments will forever be etched in my heart.

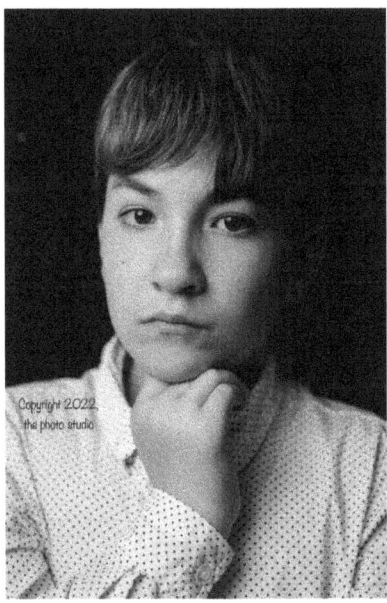

With you by my side, life feels boundless, as if it stretches on until the sun sets for the final time. This book was written with the hope that parents and caregivers who are caring for individuals with Prader-Willi Syndrome, or other types of syndromes, will gain deeper insights into this condition and the intricacies. More importantly, it aims to provide guidance on how to navigate and embrace this journey.

Aston-Martin, you may not yet realise it, but your presence has touched the lives of others through this book. I am immensely grateful for the incredible work and guidance provided by the PWS clinic medical team at the Queensland Children's Hospital. Additionally, I want to express my heartfelt appreciation to the amazing community on the Facebook page "PWS Support for Aussies." This platform has become a haven for connection, support, and a treasure trove of resources for all you incredible parents out there.

Aston-Martin you are extremely unique that your official diagnoses, as of today 15th November 2023, is Hetero-Uniparental Disomy for Chromosome 15 PWS **AND** a 1.3Megabase deletion in the Chromosome 16p.13.11 region to delete NDE1, MYH11 and several adjacent genes. A rare combination, and you are the only human on the planet with this.

With endless love,
Sebastiaan Conrad Aston-Martin Van Nuissenburg

Foreword

Life has a peculiar way of weaving unexpected threads into our journey, often leading us to places we never imagined. This book, "Rare Threads: A Life with Prader-Willi Syndrome," chronicles a deeply personal and transformative journey that began with a diagnosis and evolved into a story of resilience, love, and unwavering hope. It is about Sebastiaan van Nuissenburg's son, Aston-Martin, and the unique life they navigate together. Through this narrative, Sebastiaan aims to offer insights into living with Prader-Willi Syndrome, a condition that has profoundly shaped their lives.

The story of their journey began on a seemingly ordinary day in 2013, marked by a phone call that would change everything. As a parent, receiving news of a diagnosis like Prader-Willi Syndrome is both daunting and overwhelming as this complex genetic condition that affects many aspects of an individual's life, from physical health to emotional well-being. Suddenly, the future becomes uncertain, filled with questions and challenges that one feels ill-prepared to face. Yet, it is in these moments of uncertainty that we find our greatest strengths and discover the depths of our resilience. Aston-Martin's diagnosis was the beginning of a journey that has been both arduous and enlightening, filled with trials and triumphs that have defined their lives. Living with this condition requires a daily commitment to managing symptoms, advocating for needs, and finding joy in small victories. This book captures not only the medical and logistical aspects of managing Prader-Willi

Syndrome but also the emotional landscape that accompanies it. It is a testament to the indomitable spirit of Aston-Martin and the extraordinary love and dedication of those who support individuals with this condition.

"Rare Threads" is more than a recounting of their journey; it is a celebration of the human spirit's capacity to adapt and thrive amidst adversity. Aston-Martin's story is one of courage, perseverance, and the unwavering bond of family. It is a reminder that even in the face of significant challenges, there is always hope. Through this book, Sebastiaan seeks to empower parents, caregivers, and individuals affected by Prader-Willi Syndrome, offering a comprehensive resource that weaves together their experiences, insights, and the lessons they have learned along the way. Each chapter delves into different stages of Aston-Martin's life, highlighting the challenges they faced and the strategies they employed to overcome them. From the early years of diagnosis to navigating school and social interactions, this book provides a comprehensive look at what it means to live with Prader-Willi Syndrome. I hope that through sharing their story, others will find solace, guidance, and inspiration.

As readers journey through these pages, they are invited to walk alongside the van Nuissenburg family, to feel the weight of their struggles and the joy of their successes. May this book serve as a beacon of hope for those navigating similar paths, showcasing the unbreakable strength of love and the human spirit in the face of adversity.

Disclaimer methods

Please note that the methods presented in this book, which are based on extensive research and findings from reputable medical journals, are provided as illustrative examples for your consideration and adaptation. It is essential to recognise that these methods may not guarantee identical results for every individual or child, and adjustments may be necessary to cater to the specific needs of both parents/caregivers and participants. The information provided herein aims to offer guidance and support, but it is crucial to seek personalised advice from qualified medical professionals, as it should not serve as a substitute for their expertise.

While the author and publisher have taken great care to ensure the accuracy of the information presented in this book, they do not assume any liability for any loss, damage, or disruption caused by errors or omissions. This applies regardless of whether such errors or omissions result from negligence, accident, or any other cause.

It is strongly advised that readers regularly consult with a physician regarding their health and, particularly, any symptoms that may require diagnosis or medical attention. This book is not intended to replace the medical advice of physicians, and it is crucial to seek professional medical guidance in matters relating to one's health.

Moreover, it is important to note that the information in this book is intended to supplement, not replace, proper training in the sports mentioned in this book. Just like any sport involving speed, equipment, balance, and environmental factors, the sports mentioned carry inherent risks. Therefore, the author and publisher urge readers to assume full responsibility for their safety and to be aware of their limitations. Prior to engaging in the skills described in this book, it is essential to ensure that any equipment is well-maintained and to avoid taking risks beyond one's level of experience, aptitude, training, and comfort level.

About the Author

Sebastiaan's journey with Prader-Willi Syndrome began in 2013 when his own child was diagnosed with the condition. Motivated by a deep desire to understand and support individuals with PWS, he embarked on extensive research and conducted a comprehensive two-year case study involving his own child. This endeavour not only contributed to the advancement of PWS research but also allowed Sebastiaan to gain invaluable insights into managing this genetic disorder.

Sebastiaan Van Nuissenburg is a highly accomplished professional with a background as a former Royal Australian Navy Veteran Communication Systems Specialist. Over the course of his career, Sebastiaan has demonstrated expertise in diverse fields, including information technology, intelligence operations, and large-scale defence projects. With a Diploma of Leadership and Management, Diploma of Security Risk Management (security analysis), Diploma in Government, Psychosocial Recovery Coach short course, Advance Certificate in Sports Coaching and Nutritional Coaching, MiniRoos Certification, Special Olympics Australia – Young Athletes Coach Course, he has consistently pursued personal and professional development, enhancing his skills and knowledge.

Driven by his personal experiences and a dedication to making a positive impact, Sebastiaan developed a unique PWS program centred around creating a daily routine filled with joy and fulfillment for individuals with PWS. Now, through this book, he offers a complete and comprehensive understanding of how to effectively manage Prader-Willi Syndrome. Sebastiaan believes that the best way to truly comprehend the challenges and nuances of PWS is to immerse oneself in their world and embrace a life alongside individuals with this condition.

With a wealth of knowledge and a compassionate approach, Sebastiaan serves as a guiding voice for parents, caregivers, and professionals seeking to navigate the complexities of Prader-Willi Syndrome.

Indomitable Caregivers

If I were to stand before you in a lecture hall, or to screen to you via a webinar, this is what I would say:

Ladies and gentlemen, distinguished guests, and especially the families who are full-time carers of special needs children, I stand before you today as the author of this book to share a message of hope, resilience and the power of time management.

Life can often feel like a whirlwind, with responsibilities pulling us in every direction. We find ourselves juggling countless tasks, barely finding a moment to catch our breath.

Imagine for a moment a tightrope walker, gracefully balancing on a thin wire, defying gravity. Just like them, we too must learn to walk the tightrope of life. And in this delicate balancing act, we must find time for ourselves, for our dreams and aspirations.

In the hustle and bustle of daily life and our role as carers, we often neglect our own health. But when we find the time to exercise, even for just a few minutes each day, something magical happens. Our bodies awaken, our minds become sharper, and a renewed energy surges through our veins. Suddenly, the weight of the world feels a little lighter, and we gain the strength and resilience to face any challenge that comes our way.

In the depths of the night, when exhaustion threatens to consume us, it can be easy to lose sight of our dreams. But remember, my carer colleagues, that even the darkest hour is followed by the dawn. The road may be long, and the path may be treacherous, but with unwavering determination, we can reach the summit.

To the families who tirelessly care for their special needs children, I want you to know that your sacrifices do not go unnoticed. Your dedication, love, and perseverance are a beacon of light in a world that often overlooks the challenges you face. Your sleepless nights and tireless efforts are not in vain. You are warriors, fighting battles that many cannot comprehend.

Dear families, I implore you to find solace in the fact that you are not alone. Reach out to your support networks, lean on each other, and share your stories. Together, we can create a community that uplifts and supports one another. Remember, strength is not measured by the burdens we bear but by the courage with which we face them.

So, my friends, as we navigate the tightrope of life, remember to find time for yourself, prioritise your wellbeing, and work towards your dreams, one small goal at a time. And to the families caring for special needs children, know that you are seen, heard, and valued. Your love and dedication are shaping the future, and the world is a better place because of you.

Sebastiaan Van Nuissenburg

Rare Threads:
A Life with
Prader-Willi Syndrome

A Unique Combination of
Two Separate Genetic Conditions &
The Six Levels f Disquietude

Sebastiaan van Nuissenburg

Chapter 1

The phone call at 14:35

Thursday, August 15th, 2013, is a day that will forever be etched in my memory. At 14:35, marked a pivotal moment that altered the course of my life and everything within it. I found myself in Canberra, amidst preparations for a new job and a relocation. The plan was for me to head down first, commence work, and then shuttle back to Brisbane until the arrival of our baby. Once both my wife, Olena, and the baby were ready, we would embark on our new journey in Canberra. That day, I decided to spend some time at the zoo, soaking in the pleasant weather. As I observed the monkeys enjoying their meal, my phone rang, and the news I received changed everything. The receptionist from the medical practice in Queensland informed me that Olena had gone into labour, and an ambulance had been dispatched to take her to the hospital due to her water breaking.

I swiftly left the zoo and made my way back to a friend's place, where I was staying. I shared the unfolding events with him, and it was during this time that the realisation struck me – Olena was only thirty-six weeks into her pregnancy, far from full term. Questions and concerns flooded my mind. What could have led to this unexpected turn of events? Despite the uncertainty, I managed to secure a flight from Canberra to Brisbane within the next ninety minutes. I reached out to a friend back home, requesting him to pick me up from the airport and drive me to the hospital, to which he graciously agreed.

During the flight, my thoughts raced, attempting to decipher the reasons behind the premature birth at thirty-six weeks. I tried to find solace in the scenic views from my window seat, but my mind was a whirlwind of emotions and uncertainties. Each passing moment was filled with myriad thoughts – some hopeful, others unsettling. I found myself grappling with the unknown, unable to shake off the weight of speculation and apprehension.

When I arrived at the airport, my friend was waiting for me. As we made our way to his car, he inquired, "Which week is she in?" I responded, "Week thirty-six, which is four weeks premature." Upon reaching the hospital, my friend congratulated me and I hurried to the reception desk to inquire about Olena's whereabouts. They promptly directed me to her room. At first glance, I could see that she was in pain, but it was a different kind of pain, and the atmosphere felt heavy with unease.

Something was amiss, but it was challenging to discern exactly what. Olena expressed that she didn't feel right. At 10:00 pm, she was transferred to the labour room, and the lead midwife administered gas and instructed her to push, then gas again, followed by more pushing, in a continuous cycle. Olena questioned why she was being told to push when she didn't feel the urge or fullness to do so.

Despite Olena's evident pain, the senior midwife persisted in instructing her to push, followed by more gas, and then more pushing, for several minutes.

During Olena's challenging labour, the baby's heart rate became a cause for concern. It dropped to a worrying 57 bpm and, although it gradually increased, it remained below the normal range of 119 bpm. This unpredictable pattern persisted for over thirty minutes, creating a tense and distressing situation for me, Olena and our unborn son, Aston-Martin.

The experience was undoubtedly traumatic for Olena, and the wellbeing of the baby was at the forefront of everyone's minds. The medical team worked diligently to ensure the safety of both mother and child, and while it was a challenging time, their dedicated care helped navigate through the difficulties.

The Birth

It was at 10:26 pm that our son came into the world. As a first-time father, I was filled with a mix of emotions and uncertainties. When the midwife revealed that it was a boy, I looked down when the baby emerged. I recall there was no crying and no movements. He appeared limp, with a bluish-purplish hue, and it seemed as though he couldn't move. After being briefly placed on Olena's chest, he was quickly removed, and I had to swiftly cut the umbilical cord. The baby was then placed on a table across the room, and as the nurse held his arm, it simply flopped back onto the table without any movement.

At this precise moment, the doctor approached me and uttered words that I will never forget: "There is something wrong with your son. He is blue, not breathing properly, and appears limp. I think I know what it is." Seeing my son's arm flop back on the table and hearing the doctor's words led me to believe that our baby had not survived. He made no sound, no cries, and no movements. To me, he seemed paralysed.

The nurses immediately administered oxygen, known as CPAP, within a span of 20 to 30 seconds. A sense of panic washed over us as the nurse activated an alarm, summoning a flurry of medical personnel into the room. They swiftly moved our son into what appeared to be an incubator, surrounded by a tangle of tubes and wires. I stood frozen, grappling with a flood of questions and fears, unsure of what was unfolding before me. Olena and I were left stunned, grappling with the sudden turn of events.

After Olena had changed, the doctor approached us and suggested conducting blood tests to identify the underlying issue. We were then escorted to the Intensive Care Unit (ICU), where our son was receiving emergency treatment. Peering through the glass, I tried to gauge his condition, but the lack of information left us in a state of anguish. The waiting felt unbearable, and I struggled to maintain composure amid the uncertainty. The doctor's earlier words echoed relentlessly in my mind, overshadowing every thought and emotion.

The atmosphere was devoid of joy or reassurance; instead, it was shrouded in silence and bewilderment. We yearned for answers, for clarity, but found ourselves struggling with an overwhelming sense of helplessness. Despite my desire to seek answers from the doctor, I understood that it was too early for speculation, and that any premature conclusions could only compound our distress. It was a time fraught with emotional turmoil, leaving us clinging to hope amid the unknown.

It was a jarring revelation when I later learned that the doctor had a private conversation with Olena, disclosing his belief that our son had Prader-Willi Syndrome without the need for genetic testing, based on his prior experience. He proceeded to show her photos of his two children and to discuss the differences between his children presenting normal features when born compared to that of our son. I was unaware of this discussion at the time, but reflecting on it now, I know it would have stirred a sense of deep unease within me.

We remained at the hospital until midnight, feeling utterly drained and heavy-hearted, having been advised to go home and return the following morning. Exhausted and anxious, we faced a team of medical professionals the next day, including the head doctor, paediatrician, head nurse, and a psychologist. I braced myself for what I anticipated would be distressing news. The head doctor explained that blood tests had been conducted, but we would need to wait approximately six weeks for the results. His words weighed heavily on me, triggering a wave of anger and self-blame. I found myself immersed in irrational thoughts, questioning if I had unknowingly influenced our son's condition. The uncertainty led me to reach out to my employer in Canberra, who graciously put my employment on hold and even sent a thoughtful gesture — a plush blue teddy bear — to the hospital.

In the ensuing days, I returned to the hospital, yearning for swift answers that seemed perpetually out of reach. My son relied on tube feeding, a sight that filled me with a profound sense of helplessness. I found myself pondering his future, particularly whether he would share my passion for sports, especially soccer, where I once excelled. The six-week wait felt interminable, each day marked by a sense of longing for clarity and resolution.

When the head doctor finally delivered the test results, I greeted the word "positive" with a sense of relief, accustomed to its positive connotations in the workplace. However, I quickly learned that in the medical context, "positive" signified the opposite — unsettling news. The paediatrician and psychologist approached me, scheduling a meeting on September 24th, 2013, to delve into our son's condition and the implications of the test results. The weight of uncertainty and the impending meeting loomed over us, intensifying our yearning for understanding and guidance.

If there ever was a weekend that tested the depths of despair, it was that weekend. I found myself tossing and turning, inundated with tears and an overwhelming sense of anguish. Questions plagued my mind as I cried myself to sleep, pondering, "Why me? What have I done? Have I missed a week of church or something?"

The impending discussion

On the 12th of September, we arrived at the hospital around 5 pm, eager to see our son. As the clock neared 5:30 pm, a nurse informed us that the meeting was about to begin. We were ushered into a room where we were met by a daunting assembly of nearly ten individuals from various departments. The air was thick with apprehension; it was a meeting that defied preparation, leaving us uncertain of what to expect from each person and their respective roles. I felt a swarm of butterflies in my stomach, unease settling in as I braced myself for the impending discussion.

Each member introduced themselves, representing a spectrum of expertise including child development services from the hospital, encompassing developmental paediatricians, occupational therapists, nurses, physiotherapists, psychologists, speech pathologists, social workers, nutrition and dietetics, respiratory and sleep medicine, a genetics specialist, and the head doctor. As the head doctor began to address the gathering, I strained to absorb every word, my attention fixated on his sombre delivery. The words "Prader-Willi Syndrome" reverberated in my ears, sending shockwaves through my being. The room blurred as I dealt with the weight of this profound revelation. My mind raced, contemplating the implications for my newborn son, Aston-Martin, and the uncertain path that lay ahead.

The doctor's gentle voice carried a heavy burden as he delineated the challenges that awaited us — the relentless hunger, the developmental hurdles, the necessity for unwavering vigilance. Each word pierced me, leaving a trail of heartache in its wake. The gravity of the situation enveloped me in profound sorrow. My son, so pure and fragile, was thrust into a world fraught with adversity. The joy of his birth was now overshadowed by the daunting reality that lay before us.

I was consumed by a sense of numbness, rendered speechless and engulfed by feelings of hopelessness, shame, and profound brokenness. The question reverberated in my mind, "Why me? What have I done to deserve this?" Images of the word "syndrome" flashed through my thoughts, juxtaposed with my limited understanding and past encounters. Olena, my wife, bore the weight of the news even more heavily than I did; it hit her like a relentless freight train. The events of that night remain a hazy blur in my memory. Despite their efforts to explain, the information eluded my grasp, leaving me with fragmented recollections of the words "syndrome" and "mild."

In simpler terms, Prader-Willi Syndrome is a complex genetic disorder that manifests in myriad health, cognitive, and behavioural challenges throughout the patient's life. It stems from the lack of expression of paternal genes on chromosome 15q11.2-q13, attributed to paternal microdeletion, maternal Uniparental Disomy (UPD), or imprinting centre defects (IC). In larger populations, the likelihood stands at 1 in 30,000, and our son was one of two born that year in Queensland out of 63,837 births.

The medical team indicated that they suspected our son had Prader-Willi Syndrome, classified as mild, with the subtype being UPD, or Uniparental Disomy. This occurs when an individual inherits two chromosome copies, or part of a chromosome, from one parent and none from the other. In Aston-Martin's case, he received two chromosome copies from his mother and none from me.

My mind raced as I sought to trace back every possible factor that could have contributed to this outcome. I questioned whether my past experiences in the Navy, with my role in Communications Information & Systems and Military Intelligence, along with a highly classified security clearance, had exposed me to radiation or chemicals. I even pondered if my dietary habits or environmental factors might have played a role. My thoughts spiralled, leaving me feeling lightheaded and oppressed by the weight of the information I had just received. It felt inconceivable to reconcile this diagnosis with my lifelong commitment to sports, healthy living, and abstention from smoking or illicit substances. I found myself entertaining the fleeting notion that perhaps there had been a mix-up, and the diagnosis belonged to another child, not ours.

That night felt interminable, and as the doctor furnished me with information on Prader-Willi Syndrome, he offered a detailed account of the condition, sparing no detail. His words painted a stark picture, devoid of any semblance of sugarcoating. While he acknowledged that proper management could improve certain characteristics, he cautioned against delving into internet research, emphasising the wide spectrum of experiences within the Prader-Willi community. Each word landed heavily, underscoring the weight of the journey that lay ahead for our son and our family.

After the emotionally taxing meeting, we made our way to our son's room. I leaned in to gently kiss his forehead and whispered, "No matter what happens, you're coming home with me."

As we departed from the hospital, tears welled in my eyes, not for my own pain, but for the challenges that lay ahead for my son. I grieved for the life he might have had, for the obstacles he would inevitably confront. Yet, among the sorrow, a fierce determination took root within me. We were in this together, and we were resolved to provide our son with a life brimming with love and unwavering support. He was not merely a diagnosis — he was our son.

Every day, we returned to the hospital to spend precious moments with him. As he relied on tube feeding, the nurses patiently showed us how to carefully insert the tube through his nose and into his stomach — a procedure that was far from pleasant given his difficulty swallowing. Infants like him often exhibit signs of 'poor sucking reflex' due to diminished muscle tone, making feeding a challenging task and potentially leading to a failure to thrive.

Driven by Destiny

As the weeks passed without an official name for our son, I felt a profound desire to bestow upon him a name that was not only special, but also unforgettable. One day, while grabbing lunch across the street from the hospital, I caught sight of a distinctive sports car that exuded elegance and sophistication. It immediately brought to mind the iconic 007 James Bond and his association with the renowned Aston Martin. I felt that a remarkable boy with extraordinary strength deserved a name that echoed his uniqueness.

Upon researching the history of Aston Martin, I discovered that the company was incorporated in 1913 by Lionel Martin and Robert Bamford. Fast forward 100 years to 2013, and it seemed to me the perfect way to name a truly special child. I named him ASTON-MARTIN, a name that resonated with significance and held a personal connection as it bore a resemblance to my father's name, Anton Martinus. Upon returning to the hospital, I initiated the name application process, sharing my idea with Olena. While she agreed, her expression conveyed a blend of understanding and puzzlement — a classic case of the enigmatic ways of women!

Daily, we made our way back to the hospital, where we eagerly participated in Aston-Martin's tube feeding, cradled him in our arms, and revelled in the precious moments when he would open his eyes and bless us with his heartwarming smile. During infancy, one of the primary indicators to watch for is poor muscle tone, known as hypotonia. Babies with this condition may appear limp, with loosely extended elbows and knees, resembling rag dolls when held. Aston-Martin exhibited these characteristics, making it feel like I was holding a delicate, life-sized doll in my arms. Additionally, distinct facial features such as almond-shaped eyes, a downturned mouth, and a thin upper lip were noticeable. He seemed unusually tired, had a weak cry, and slept extensively, prompting concerns that led to his three-month stay in the ICU.

Nasogastric Tube

The most notable aspect of our caregiving journey was the process of nasogastric tube (NG tube) feeding. It was indeed a daunting experience, as Aston-Martin faced challenges in properly suckling and lacked the necessary strength to do so. Our attempts to feed him through a bottle equipped with a small nipple often proved arduous, prompting us to explore alternative methods. One such approach involved thickening the breast milk and administering it on a spoon, gently urging it against his lips so that his tongue could take the lead in the feeding process. While this method yielded gradual progress, it remained essential for him to develop the ability to suck. This significant undertaking continued for a period of three months, with daily visits for feeding sessions and guidance on NG tube management.

The initial stages of learning how to insert the tube were disconcerting, as the sensation was far from pleasant, and the fear of inadvertently causing discomfort or, worse, inserting the tube into his airway loomed large. With reassurance from the nurses, I persevered, albeit cautiously, as it became increasingly likely that Aston-Martin would require an NG tube upon returning home. Furthermore, tending to his positioning in the cot became exclusively my responsibility, as he was unable to adjust himself. This realisation brought with it a tinge of sadness, compounded by the unexpected nature of our extended hospital stay. These assorted challenges gradually took a toll on my emotional wellbeing, and coming to terms with this new reality proved mentally taxing.

However, amidst these challenges, there were unexpected glimmers of hope. Aston-Martin defied expectations by no longer requiring tube feeding and exhibiting early signs of independent movement, a remarkable feat that surprised the medical team. Typically, infants do not display such mobility until they are eighteen months or older, yet Aston-Martin achieved this milestone in just three months.

Further surprises awaited us during his eye examination. Despite the likelihood of poor eyesight and the anticipated need for prescription glasses, the ophthalmologist was astonished to discover that Aston-Martin had perfect vision. Incredulous, he sought a second opinion from the head ophthalmologist, who confirmed the astonishing results. As I pondered this unforeseen turn of events, I found myself entertaining the notion of a guardian angel watching over my son, or perhaps even considering the possibility of a misdiagnosis. The doctor emphasised that the odds of a misdiagnosis were extremely rare, akin to a one-in-a-million chance.

After a long and arduous three months at the hospital, the time finally arrived to bring Aston-Martin home. We spent an additional night in a private room at the hospital, attentively learning how to assist him with movement and proper feeding, as well as receiving essential first-aid instructions. These three months were merely the prologue to the journey that lay ahead, and I wondered with uncertainty about what the future held. Despite the trials and tribulations, my world was forever changed for the better.

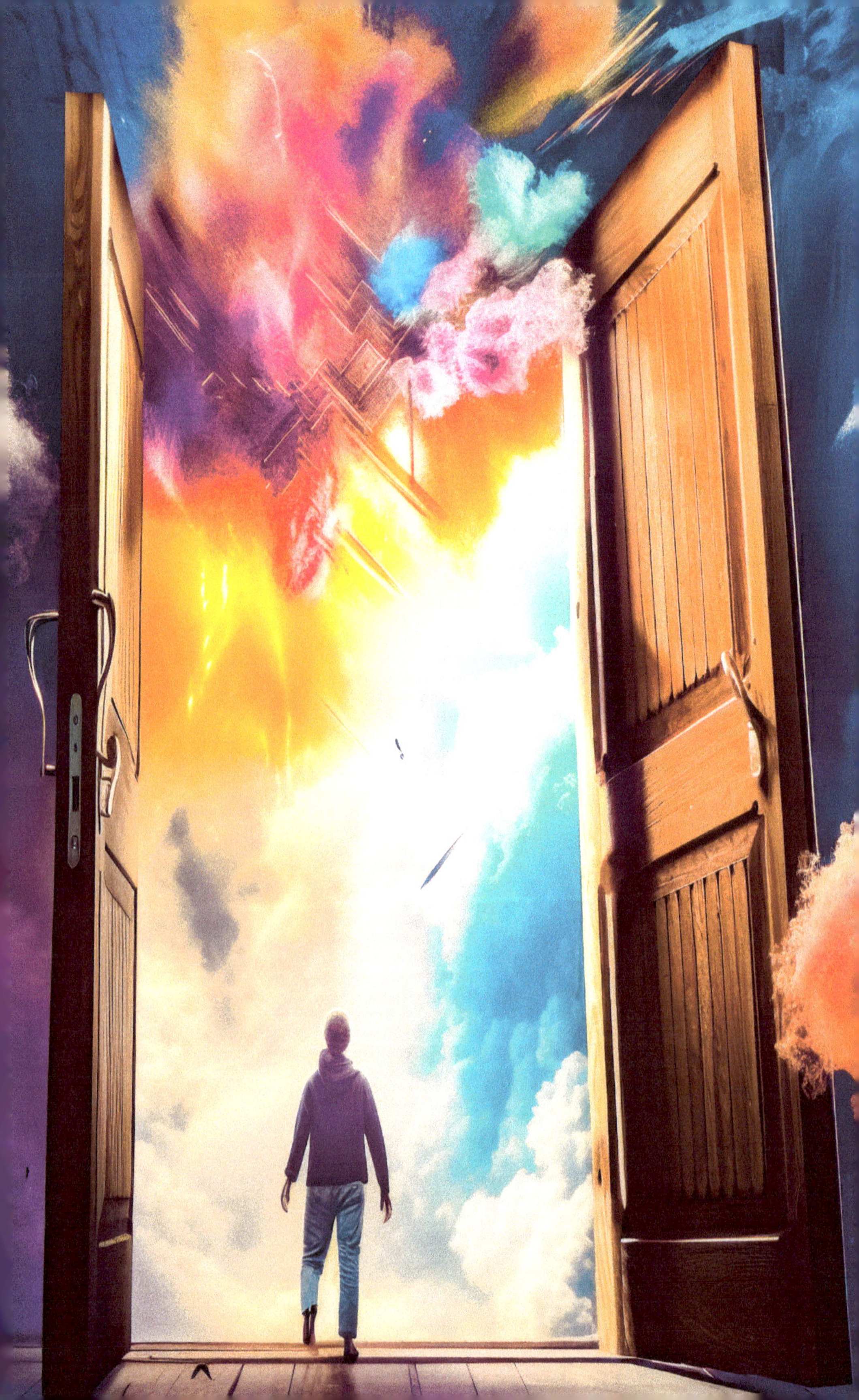

Chapter 2

A World of Challenges and Uncertain Magic

In the dimly lit doctor's office, the weight of the diagnosis hung heavy in the air, suffocating Sebastiaan's heart with fear and uncertainty. The doctor's words had twisted and contorted into a monstrous form, clawing at his very core. The revelation of Prader-Willi Syndrome had shattered their world, leaving them adrift in a sea of unknowns.

Sebastiaan's gaze faltered, unable to meet the doctor's solemn eyes. His son, Aston-Martin, lay peacefully in his crib, unaware of the storm raging around him. The doctor's voice pierced the silence, each word a dagger to Sebastiaan's soul.

"Prader-Willi Syndrome, as you know from our previous meeting, is what your son Aston-Martin has been officially diagnosed with," the doctor's voice trembled with gravity, " and is a rare condition, one that will require unwavering strength and infinite love from you, Sebastiaan. It's a journey fraught with challenges and uncertainty but one that can be faced with courage."

Sebastiaan's hands clenched into fists, his breaths shallow and uneven. The weight of his son's future bore down on him with crushing intensity. But amid the darkness, a flicker of determination ignited within him.

"I will do whatever it takes," Sebastiaan's voice shook with raw emotion, his eyes finally meeting the doctor's gaze. "Aston-Martin is my son, and I will walk this path with him, no matter how daunting, I'll find out as much as I can and try to work around this Prader-Willi Syndrome."

The doctor's expression softened, a glimmer of hope shining through the sombre atmosphere. "You are stronger than you know, Sebastiaan. Your love for Aston-Martin will guide you through the darkest of times."

Aston-Martin stirred in his sleep, a soft hum escaping his lips. Sebastiaan's resolve solidified, a newfound strength coursing through his veins. In that moment, amidst the echoes of fear and uncertainty, a bond between father and son grew unbreakable.

As they left the doctor's office, the weight of the diagnosis remained heavy on Sebastiaan's shoulders, but he carried it with newfound purpose and determination. The journey ahead would be arduous, but with love as their shield, they would face it head-on, united in their unyielding resolve.

If this were a work of fiction, it would read something like that. Sadly, this is a true story and reads more as follows.

The journey with Prader-Willi Syndrome is akin to stepping into a world of unknown spells and unpredictable potions. Every day presents a unique set of challenges, each demanding its own brand of magic to navigate. From managing the relentless hunger to tackling the complex behavioural symptoms, it is a constant dance of adaptation and innovation.

The hunger, an ever-present force, requires vigilant management. It is a battle against the body's own dark magic, where cravings can lead to excessive weight gain and health complications. The solution lies in a delicate balance of nutrition and portion control, a dietary spell book crafted by experts. Every meal becomes a carefully calculated creation, a culinary enchantment designed to satisfy without fuelling the insatiable hunger.

Behavioural challenges add another layer of complexity to this already enigmatic condition. The mood swings and temperamental shifts can be as unpredictable as a wand choosing its wizard. One moment, we are sailing smoothly through calm waters; the next, we are navigating turbulent seas, requiring all hands on deck to weather the storm.

The quest for growth hormones is yet another adventure in this PWS journey. These precious potions, when administered correctly, hold the key to unlocking Aston-Martin's full potential. They are the elixir that supports his development, but their continued use relies on maintaining a healthy weight. It is a delicate dance, for any excess weight gain could mean forfeiting access to these vital treatments.

In this world of PWS, nothing can be taken for granted. Every aspect of our lives must be carefully curated to support Aston-Martin's needs. Social interactions require careful planning, for the potential triggers are myriad. From the food served at gatherings to the understanding of those around us, every detail must be considered to ensure Aston-Martin's comfort and safety.

As Aston-Martin grows and evolves, so does the nature of the challenges. His cognitive development takes unexpected turns, demanding constant re-evaluation and adaptation. It is as though we are deciphering an ancient language, learning to interpret his unique expressions and gestures, his own form of communication.

The support network we cultivate becomes our fortress. From therapists to educators, each brings their own brand of sorcery to help us navigate this enchanted journey. They offer strategies and insights, guiding us through the maze of symptoms and providing tools to empower Aston-Martin to conquer his challenges.

In this world, there are no guarantees, no clear-cut paths to follow. Each person with PWS writes their own unique story, and it is our duty to provide the love, support, and resources they need to flourish. It is a journey of self-discovery, resilience, and the unwavering belief in the magic that lies within us all.

As we continue on this path, we embrace the unknown, knowing that each step brings us closer to unlocking the mysteries of Prader-Willi Syndrome. Together, we face the challenges, celebrate the victories, and cherish the unique gifts that Aston-Martin brings into our lives. It is a journey of endurance, courage, and above all, a testament to the power of unconditional love.

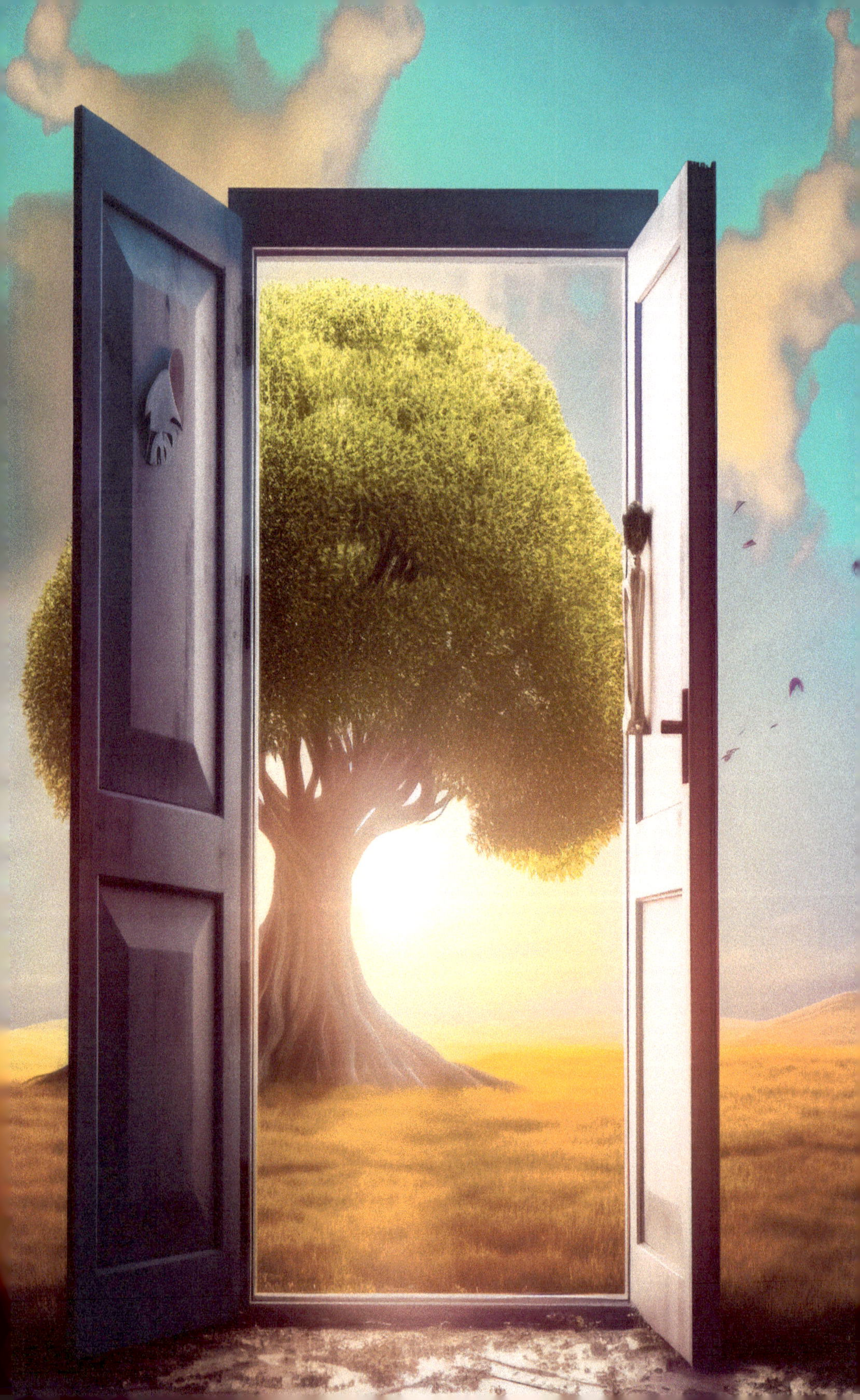

CHAPTER 3

Taking on the Journey

Finally, Aston-Martin was home, and a new chapter of our lives had begun. We nestled him in a cosy baby cot, and the journey ahead seemed both daunting and filled with hope. The initial twelve months brought a blend of ease and challenges. On the one hand, the absence of hyperphagia, or excessive hunger and food-seeking behaviour, offered a sense of relief. We carefully provided him with the appropriate amount of food, ensuring his weight remained within the normal range, despite his small size. Surprisingly, he rarely cried, granting us peaceful nights and ample opportunities for rest. Tasks such as changing him and giving him a bath also proved to be relatively effortless.

It was the numerous appointments that posed a significant challenge. Spread across a gruelling five-day schedule, Aston-Martin's week included three physiotherapy appointments, two occupational therapy sessions, and a general practitioner visit. Each child with Prader-Willi Syndrome receives tailored care based on the severity of their condition. Additionally, he had two hospital appointments per month, along with biannual visits to the Prader-Willi clinic at the children's hospital. Over the course of his first twelve months, he underwent a staggering 156 physiotherapy appointments to help him build strength and develop essential motor skills, given his hypotonia.

Aston-Martin's journey also benefitted from the support of a federally funded program designed to assist families with children diagnosed with disabilities — the 'Better Start Initiative'. This initiative provided approximately twelve-thousand dollars to aid in Aston-Martin's care and development until the age of seven, offering significant assistance during this formative period.

The physiotherapists' understanding and flexibility were invaluable, as they offered us a discounted rate and were understanding of any necessary cancellations. Without this program, I would have struggled to secure the financial means to continue Aston-Martin's essential physiotherapy sessions, crucial for his development given his condition. The initiative granted us access to a wide array of professionals, including psychologists, a speech pathologist, occupational therapist, audiologist, optometrist, orthoptist, and physiotherapist, providing comprehensive support for Aston-Martin's diverse needs.

These appointments, each lasting an hour and scheduled either in the morning or midday, necessitated a significant time commitment, with approximately two hours of travel time for each session. Balancing the demands of caring for a special needs child with a full-time job proved to be unfeasible, prompting me to step back from the workforce. Fortunately, my previous experience as a contractor in defence, working in information technology with a high-level security clearance, had allowed me to accumulate substantial savings. While this financial cushion provided some relief, it was clear that these resources needed to be allocated primarily for Aston-Martin's needs, given the uncertainty of what lay ahead.

The occupational therapist's guidance, with sessions twice a week, proved to be instrumental, as they focused on enhancing Aston-Martin's fine motor skills, decision-making abilities, and learning new skills. Initially, Aston-Martin viewed the sessions as a game, but as the therapist worked with him, I also learned valuable techniques that I could implement at home. Visual learning suited me best, and I diligently observed and replicated the therapist's methods, ensuring that we could continue the learning process within our home environment.

Similarly, I actively participated in Aston-Martin's physiotherapy sessions, attending as many as possible to grasp the techniques and implement them at home. Embracing a hands-on approach, I procured the same toys used during his therapy sessions, using them to further his development. Starting with simple building blocks, we observed his progress as he gradually mastered the task.

Watching Aston-Martin struggle with his coordination was a challenge, yet there was a sense that he was trying to emulate me, his daddy. Despite his determination, his coordination remained a hurdle, causing him to frequently knock over the coloured blocks we used for learning. Our goal was to encourage him to stack blocks of the same colour, starting with blue blocks, and patiently guiding him as he attempted to replicate my actions. It was a slow process for him to grasp, especially given his limited language skills, rendering spoken words as mere gibberish to him. English, the language around him, was like a foreign tongue, its meaning and nuances beyond his reach.

Our routine included regular visits to the general practitioner, typically scheduled once every fortnight on Fridays, to assess Aston-Martin's progress. These appointments, lasting fifteen to twenty minutes, involved measurements of his height, weight, head circumference, and waist circumference. It became evident that his physical development deviated from that of his peers, with his short stature and slight overweight attributed to his slow metabolism, resulting in an inability to efficiently process energy. These appointments, combined with the multitude of therapy sessions, amounted to a staggering 288 appointments within the first year, a number that felt overwhelming and exhausting.

Caring for a special needs child became a full-time commitment, surpassing the demands of raising a typically developing child. Although Aston-Martin's quiet nature made certain tasks more manageable, it also meant missing out on the typical expressions and interactions that accompany a child's vocalisations. Finding social groups for him proved to be a challenge, as the available options were primarily located at special schools, which he was still too young to attend. We had to patiently wait until he turned three before exploring these opportunities further.

At nine months of age, we had our upcoming appointment at the children's hospital with the lead paediatrician held a familiar sense of comfort, as she had been involved in Aston-Martin's care since his birth. I confided in her about the challenges of finding work from home employment while caring for a special needs child, and she kindly suggested exploring childcare centres as a potential solution. Eager to explore this option, I reached out to a centre in a nearby suburb only to be met with a disheartening response. The abrupt dismissal of Aston-Martin's needs left me speechless, as the lady on the other end of the line bluntly stated that they did not cater to "those kind" of children. The call ended with a sense of shock and disbelief, leaving me to grapple with the unfair judgment imposed on my son without even meeting him.

Meanwhile, the paediatrician informed me that Aston-Martin's upcoming medication would necessitate a sleep study, and we promptly arranged the appointment over the phone. Upon sharing my disheartening experience with the paediatrician, she expressed her disbelief and reassured me that the process of enlisting allied health support at a childcare centre was straightforward, involving simple documentation to be submitted to the Queensland Health Department. She promptly emailed me the necessary forms, and I wasted no time in printing them out, eager to explore every avenue to ensure Aston-Martin's wellbeing and inclusion.

Determined to secure a supportive environment for Aston-Martin, I arranged a meeting at another nearby childcare centre, hopeful that a face-to-face discussion might lead to a positive outcome. I candidly explained my son's condition, Prader-Willi Syndrome, and the necessity of one-to-one supervision, emphasising the availability of an allied health worker at no cost to the centre.

Despite my efforts to convey the importance of individualized care, the centre director seemed disinterested in the allied health documents I brought. Her demeanour spoke volumes, and while she expressed willingness to accept Aston-Martin, she made it clear that they might not always be able to provide the level of supervision he required. As we conversed, I observed Aston-Martin navigating the play equipment, only to witness him lose his balance and fall from a raised cubby house. It was a stark reminder of his struggle to comprehend depth, and as I hurried to comfort him, I couldn't shake off the unease of leaving him in a setting that failed to acknowledge his specific needs, despite the potential support of allied health professionals.

The realisation that childcare centres were either unable or unwilling to accommodate our needs or dismissed the idea due to paperwork concerns was disheartening. It was clear that the prospect of an allied health worker's involvement from the Queensland Government made the centres reluctant to proceed with the support. On the drive home, I pondered the unfairness of the situation. The looming challenge of securing a support worker while working became increasingly daunting, as their full-day payment would consume my entire salary, leaving little to cover essential expenses.

The hospital's assessment that Aston-Martin required round-the-clock care added to our stress, leaving us with the difficult decision of having one parent stay at home while the other worked. While this arrangement provided some relief, navigating the

Australian Government's social security system, referred to as Services Australia or Centrelink, proved to be an additional hurdle. Securing the carer's allowance, while helpful, fell short of meeting our needs, leaving us hopeful for a smoother process when Aston-Martin becomes eligible for the disability support pension in the future. This journey has been filled with challenges, but our hope and determination to provide the best care for Aston-Martin remain unwavering.

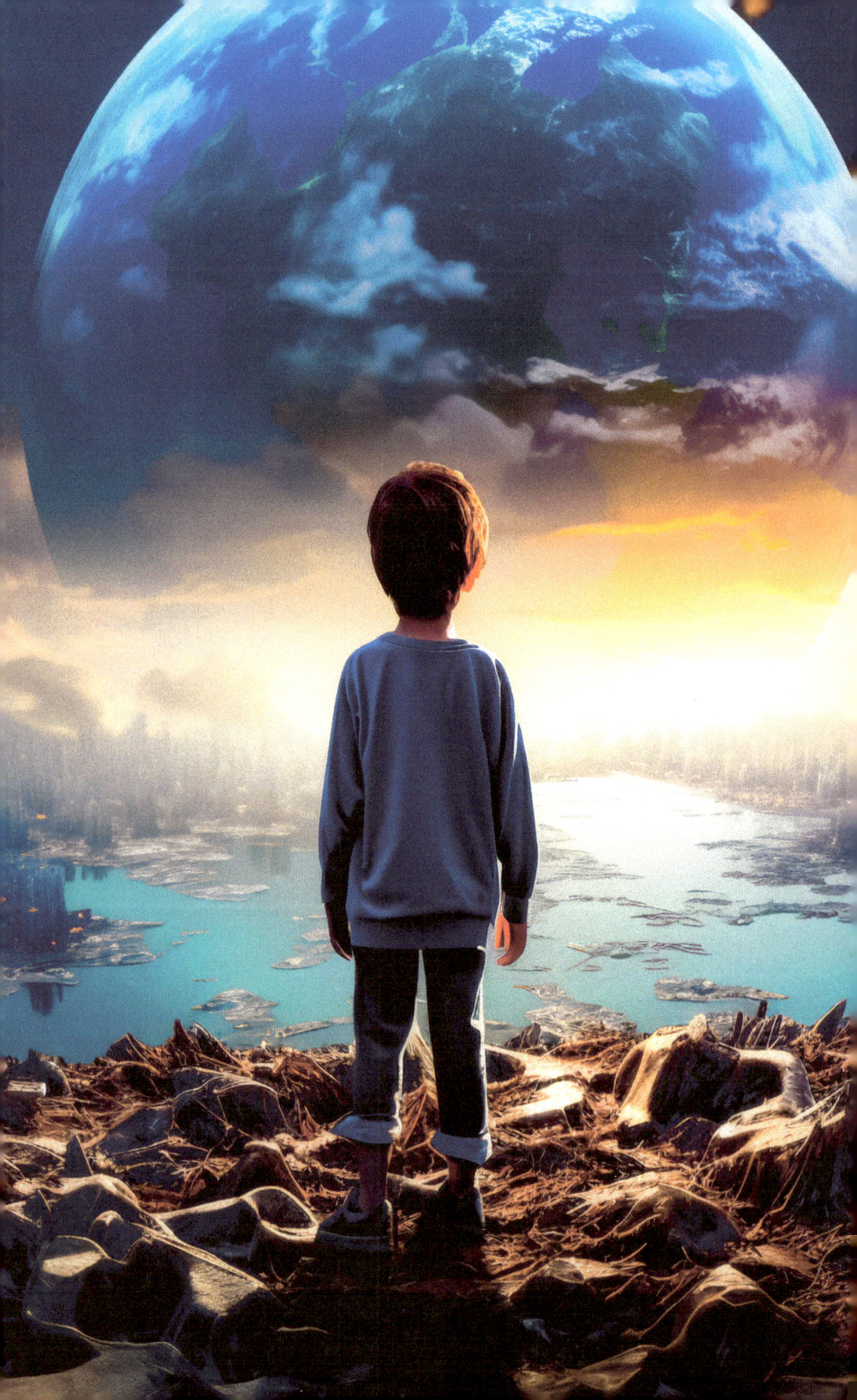

Chapter 4

Early Years and Growing Challenges – Age One

As Aston-Martin's first birthday approached, it marked a significant milestone in his life, a celebration of reaching twelve months. His birthday was a joyous occasion, and at this stage, the telltale signs of hyperphagia, the insatiable appetite, were not yet apparent. However, we noticed Aston's occasional attempts to grab anything within reach and place it in his mouth, a subtle indication of an increasing interest in food. Over time, this inclination grew, and the doctors cautioned us that the true onset of food-seeking behaviour typically begins at the age of two.

Following his first birthday, our routine of appointments continued, with the addition of a sleep study requirement. This meant that in preparation for commencing growth hormone therapy, which involved a daily injection in the thigh, Aston-Martin had to stay at the hospital for monitoring of his sleeping patterns. The growth hormone injections, known as Genotropin by Pfizer, were a financial relief, as they were included in the Australian Government's Pharmaceutical Benefit Scheme (PBS), which subsidises expensive medications. I discovered that if I were to purchase these injections directly from the United States, the annual cost would amount to $34,000, excluding additional expenses for special airfreight. The financial burden was further compounded by the costs of private physiotherapy, occupational therapy, and speech pathology services, totalling $74,000 for the first twelve months of Aston-Martin's life. However, the inclusion of the growth hormone injections under the PBS significantly alleviated our financial strain, reducing our out-of-pocket expenses to $40,760. He was on a $12,000 Better Start Initiative which helped, until the National Disability Insurance Scheme (NDIS) came into effect. This would be the following year, we hoped, but he was on the wait list, so it was just a waiting game.

The sleep study appointment was a significant milestone. Aston-Martin spent the night at the hospital while his brain wave activity, particularly in REM sleep, was meticulously recorded. The intricacies of sleep stages were explained to us, from non-rapid eye movement (NREM) to rapid eye movement (REM) sleep, each with its distinct characteristics. Aston-Martin's sleep cycle and REM stage were closely monitored, as his growth hormone injections were to be tailored based on his sleep study report, considering the energy consumption during sleep.

At one year and ten months, just before turning two, Aston-Martin commenced the medication, with a scheduled review after six weeks to assess its impact on his sleep patterns. The subsequent review revealed that the growth hormone was exerting a significant toll on his energy levels during sleep, prompting the doctor to advise discontinuing the medication to prevent potential health issues. It was a bewildering moment for me, as I struggled to fully grasp the technical details, but the gravity of the situation was clear: the medication was taking a heavy toll on Aston-Martin's wellbeing during sleep. The decision to cease the growth hormone was made, with the understanding that this space would be revisited at a later time, pending another sleep review in twelve months.

Navigating the complexities of Aston-Martin's medical care has been a journey filled with emotional highs and lows, and this experience underscored the importance of closely monitoring and responding to his unique needs. Our unwavering commitment to his wellbeing remained at the forefront of every decision, and we continued to navigate this journey with love, determination, and a profound hope for the future.

The process of applying a growth hormone is incredibly meticulous. Any missteps, such as inaccuracies in weight, height, or missed appointments at the genetics department, can lead to the PBS halting the provision of the growth hormone. As Aston-Martin was off this medication due to the potential health concerns, he missed out on growth stimulation, affecting his metabolism and leading to weight gain. This posed a significant challenge for our family, particularly for Aston-Martin.

We had to intensify his daily exercises and sports activities to support his metabolism. Our refrigerator remained stocked with organic foods and fruits, ensuring that if Aston-Martin reached for something, it wouldn't pose a risk to his health. The time had come for our son to undergo another sleep study to assess the possibility of resuming treatment. After staying overnight at the hospital, we returned to review the results with the doctor, who ultimately reapproved his treatment. The process of obtaining the growth hormone back in 2016 was arduous and protracted, involving multiple steps from script requests to medication retrieval, each demanding careful attention and time.

After resuming the growth hormone treatment, Aston-Martin's next appointment was scheduled six weeks later and, this time, the review yielded positive results, with the doctor advising us to continue as normal. About a month into the treatment, we noticed a slight decrease in his weight and a small increase in his height, signalling that we were back on track.

The journey has been undeniably challenging, with the relentless cycle of appointments and sleep studies taking its toll. There were days when the weight of it all made me long for a break, a chance to escape and recharge.

Reflecting on Aston-Martin's first birthday, I knew that we had one year left before the onset of hyperphagia, a progression that would bring about significant changes. I delved into extensive research on Prader-Willi Syndrome, immersing myself in medical journals to gain a deeper understanding of this rare genetic condition, which affects only a small number of individuals in Australia and globally. The more I delved into these journals, the more engrossing it became, providing valuable insights into potential clinical trials, tests, and medications. This knowledge empowered me with a clearer understanding of what to expect, serving as a vital guide through this complex journey.

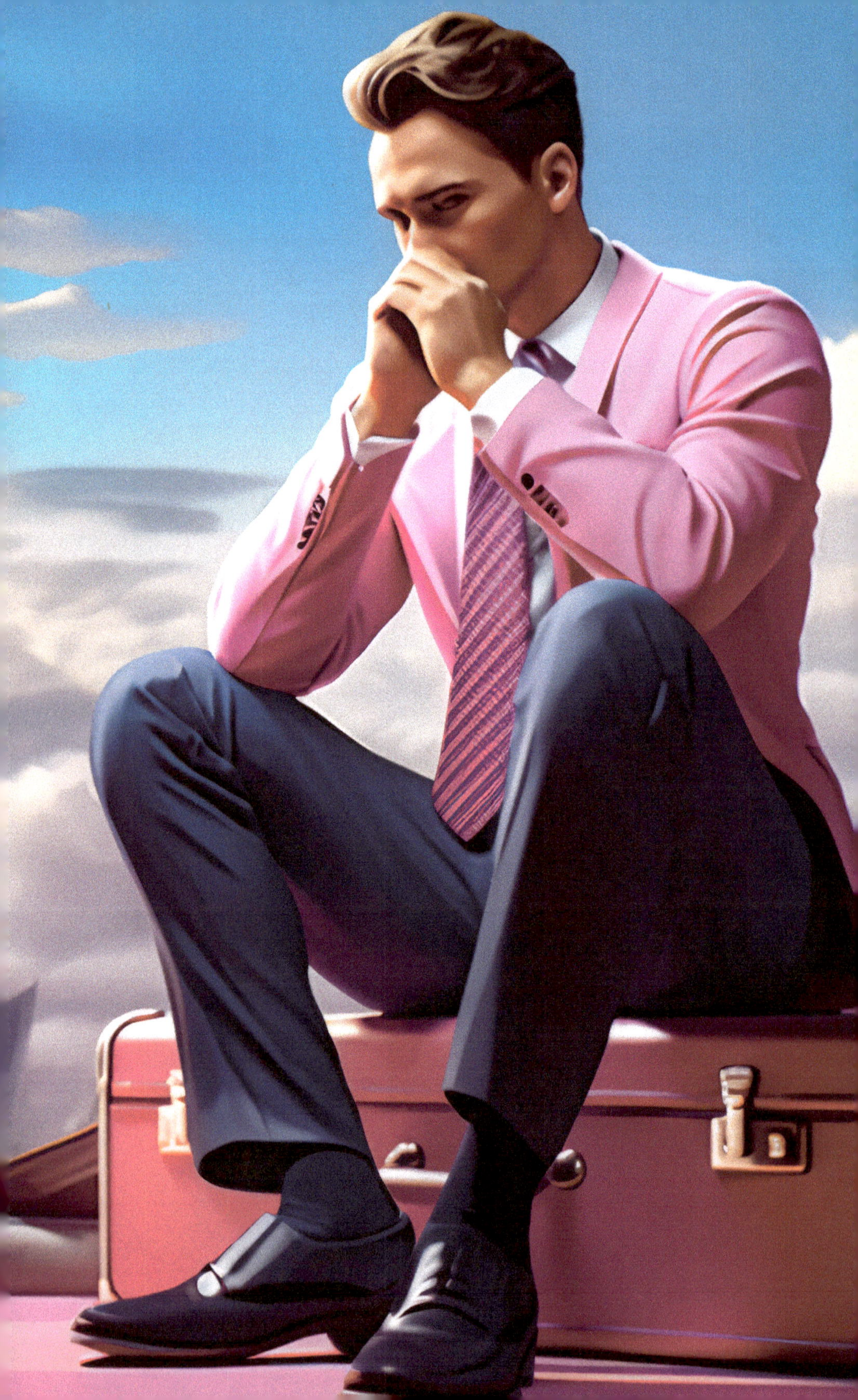

Chapter 5

Coping Strategies and Adjustments – Age Two

Aston-Martin's second birthday was a joyous occasion, filled with laughter, love, and a delicious cake from the cheesecake shop. We spent the day at Noosa, enjoying the beach, swimming, and basking in the warm sun. It was truly the best day ever!

As Aston-Martin turned two, I had already mentally prepared myself for the changes that lay ahead. I knew that it would require a complete overhaul of my lifestyle, presenting a formidable challenge as I navigated moments of potential regression. Up until the age of two, behavioural issues are not prominently noticeable, but they gradually begin to surface. The first signs emerged as Aston-Martin started grabbing and attempting to taste various items.

I vividly recall the doctors' advice to only have toys that were larger than twice the size of his hands, ensuring that they couldn't be placed in his mouth. Yet, he would grab everything from toys and blankets to leaves and dirt, demonstrating an insatiable curiosity. This behaviour extended beyond toys, encompassing personal items and household objects throughout different rooms. These early experiences served as a preparation for what was to come, offering insights into what to expect and how to manage it, as the challenges truly intensified from two-and-a-half to three years of age.

The challenges that await when dealing with the onset of PWS are immense. As a parent, you will grapple with feelings of bewilderment, frustration, anxiety and anger, emotions that are difficult to prepare for if you've never encountered this condition before. It's a journey that leaves you feeling lost and isolated, unsure of what to do or expect.

Managing the emotional turmoil experienced by children with PWS is a daunting task. These children struggle to regulate their emotions, often experiencing heightened anxiety and stress. Learning to recognise the warning signs of emotional distress, often manifested as meltdowns, is crucial. Understanding the triggers behind these meltdowns is key to managing their behaviour, but it's not an easy feat. The children are steadfast in their belief that they are right, and you are wrong, adding an extra layer of complexity to the situation.

The focal point of PWS is hyperphagia, the relentless drive to eat excessively. This insatiable appetite is active around the clock and often leads to temper outbursts, causing further anxiety and stress for the child. Managing this aspect proved to be incredibly challenging in the beginning. There were moments when I felt utterly overwhelmed, as though my heart had sunk to the depths of the earth. It was crucial to remind myself that it wasn't his fault; this was the result of a genetic abnormality with no simple solution. Early intervention in managing the child's relationship with food is paramount, teaching them portion control and the proper use of measuring cups to instil an understanding of appropriate serving sizes.

Navigating the complexities of managing PWS demands unwavering patience, understanding, and a commitment to nurturing a supportive environment for the child's wellbeing.

Making adjustments to our eating habits became a vital part of managing Aston-Martin's condition. It was crucial to prioritise healthier eating, as the risk of obesity could lead to a cascade of medical issues that spiralled out of control, potentially jeopardising his wellbeing.

Implementing a structured approach to his diet involved maintaining regular mealtimes, steering clear of sugary and high-calorie snacks, and serving smaller portions of carbohydrates. Aston-Martin's insatiable hunger made self-regulation impossible, necessitating us to take measures such as locking cupboards and the fridge, and ensuring that food remained out of sight and out of reach.

I vividly remember the day I locked the fridge with a padlock. Aston-Martin tried in vain to open it, his frustration palpable as he tugged at the handle, shaking the fridge in his determination. It was a moment that filled me with a sense of unease, fearing that the fridge might tip over.

Teaching Aston-Martin about portion sizes was another crucial aspect of managing his diet. Using medium-sized cereal bowls and the metric cup proved to be instrumental in guiding his understanding of serving sizes. It was essential we demonstrated to and involved him in the process to instil a sense of familiarity and routine. Selecting cereals with a minimum rating of 3.5 stars became a priority, ensuring that we chose from the healthiest options available to support his nutritional needs.

These adjustments were not just about managing his diet; they were a vital part of creating a supportive environment to safeguard Aston-Martin's health and wellbeing.

Let me share with you some insights about nutrition and its vital role in managing Aston-Martin's condition. Whole grains are truly nutritional powerhouses, encompassing the full spectrum of the grain's layers, from the fibre-rich outer bran to the nutrient-rich germ and the starchy endosperm. Their high fibre content is crucial, aiming for at least 10 grams per 100 grams to support a healthy gut and sustain a feeling of fullness, which can be particularly challenging with PWS children, as they struggle to recognise when they are full. Additionally, it's essential to prioritise options low in added sugar, targeting less than 15 grams per 100 grams, and low in saturated fat.

In our quest for suitable breakfast drinks, I found that using coconut water for Aston-Martin not only aided in hydration but also served as a natural laxative, promoting easier digestion.

Embracing these nutritional guidelines became a cornerstone of our routine, serving as a vital tool in managing Aston-Martin's weight. We were acutely aware of the dangers of overeating, which can lead to weight gain, obesity, and a host of associated health issues. In the context of PWS, the inability to recognise fullness poses a heightened risk, potentially leading to serious complications such as gastric perforation, a condition where overeating can result in a full-thickness injury of the stomach wall, posing a grave threat to health.

Understanding the implications of gastric perforation has been a sobering aspect of managing Aston-Martin's condition. In cases of acute perforation, the absence of an inflammatory response leaves the gastric contents free to enter the peritoneal cavity, leading to chemical peritonitis. Conversely, perforations occurring over a prolonged period may be contained locally by the body's inflammatory reaction. Suspecting perforation hinges on the patient's clinical presentation, and confirmation often arises from diagnostic imaging that reveals extraluminal free air, typically performed to investigate abdominal pain or other symptoms. The gravity of the situation is underscored by the necessity of surgical repair as the primary treatment approach. To us, this underscored the vital importance of meticulous food management in ensuring Aston-Martin's survival. Below is a short article written by Marisa Wexler, who holds a Master of Science in cellular and molecular pathology from the University of Pittsburgh, where she studied novel genetic drivers of ovarian cancer. Her areas of expertise include cancer biology, immunology, and genetics, and she has worked as a science writer as an intern for the Genetics Society of America.

Little is known about whether there is any direct connection between hyperphagia and PWS-related morbidity/mortality, outside of the indirect connection due to obesity. A quintet of scientists at the University of Cambridge in the U.K. conducted a review of published scientific studies to better understand these relationships.

In total, the team reviewed 110 studies, most of which were from relatively affluent countries such as the U.S., Japan, Australia, and several nations in Europe. Mortality data suggested that the average age of death for PWS patients was about 22 years.

From the studies, the team identified 500 cases where a person with PWS died from a known cause. The majority of these patients were obese, and the most common causes of death — such as breathing and heart problems — have well-established connections with obesity. However, in addition to these common obesity-linked causes of death, a smaller number of patients died due to choking (dysphagia) (30 patients), drowning in the bath (4 patients), or accidents (18 patients).

The most challenging part of this journey has been coming to terms with the sobering statistic that the average life expectancy for individuals with PWS is 22 years. Recognising that obesity is the leading cause of mortality, with other deaths stemming from obesity-related complications, we set out to diligently manage Aston-Martin's food intake and preventing obesity — and we have been able to extend his life expectancy by several years, if not decades. However, it's an ongoing commitment that demands unwavering dedication and vigilance. Giving up is not an option. Without proactive management, the stark reality is that PWS mortality is indeed capped at 22 years.

Incorporating physical activity into Aston-Martin's regimen assumed a pivotal role in our intervention approach. Pursuing an

Advanced Certificate in Sports and Nutritional Coaching equipped me with the knowledge and tools necessary to coach Aston-Martin, resulting in a substantial reduction in his weight. Although he remains marginally overweight, it is a manageable situation, and I am adept at handling it with minimal complications.

My primary concern revolved not so much around his dietary habits, as we successfully managed this aspect through the organisation of our refrigerator, but rather his dysphagia and the potential risk of choking during meals. We observed that he tended to stuff his mouth excessively, to the extent that his food seemed poised to escape from his palate. Upon observing his chewing habits, it became evident that he lacked the sensory awareness to cough, swallow properly, or expel food if it proved too large. This indicated a high risk of choking, as the lack of coordination in swallowing increases the likelihood of dysphagia

The impending risk of choking prompted me to anticipate the need for the Heimlich manoeuvre. I took it upon myself to carefully portion any items on his plate that I recognised as potentially hazardous to him. The issue primarily stemmed from his inadequate chewing and tendency to swallow large portions whole.

As a result, I commenced a practice of cutting his food into smaller pieces and demonstrated proper chewing techniques. In certain instances, I even pre-chewed the meat for him, similar to how a mother bird would provide food for its young. During every meal – breakfast, lunch, and dinner – I emphasised the importance of chewing and encouraged him to slow down before swallowing. I made it a point to be present during his meals to continually remind him to chew. Additionally, I instructed him to take small sips of his drink while chewing to aid in softening the food and facilitating its passage down the throat.

On top of this, it appeared that Aston-Martin approached every meal as a race, consuming his food hurriedly. I endeavoured to convey to him the importance of savouring his meals and taking his time while eating. I provided a straw for every beverage he consumed, as this aids in coordinating the swallowing process. Through this practice, he began to comprehend the mechanics of swallowing and effectively exercised the coordination aspect.

From the age of two, I implemented various cues to assist him in swallowing, many of which are self-explanatory and common knowledge, with supervision being the most crucial. I share the following key lessons we learned:

Supervision While Eating: It's important for the child to be closely monitored during meals to ensure they're chewing properly and not taking too large bites, as they might not recognise when they are full or may have a desire to eat quickly. Continuous prompting is required to help them slow down and chew more before swallowing.

Consistency of Food: Pureed or soft foods might be easier to swallow. Avoid hard, sticky, or very fibrous foods that can be hard to chew and swallow. Spaghetti is a favourite, and pasta, but I make sure we cut up the pasta prior to serving so it is easier to chew and swallow. So, choosing the foods is a must.

Small Bites: Encourage small bites and portion food appropriately to prevent the child from trying to eat too much at once. Each plate we have is the same size, and I portion out the foods on his plate evenly, and cut up anything that is required.

Chew Thoroughly: Teach and remind the child to chew their food thoroughly before swallowing. Constant cues are required to help them to chew more.

Eating Slowly: Encourage the child to eat slowly, which can be facilitated by using utensils like small spoons or forks to limit the amount of food in each bite. I usually have YouTube playing on the tv as our son eats, and I noticed he slows down when watching his kids shows. This is a strategy that works for him, and even though it's not the best, as meals times are more about family, it saves him in the long term.

Proper Seating Position: Ensure the child is seated in an upright position, ideally at a 90-degree angle, during and for at least 30 minutes after eating to help with swallowing. Upon finishing his meals, I encourage our son to stay at the dinner table and watch via the iPad his Kids YouTube channel for at least thirty minutes so he maintains the correct upright seating position.

Swallowing Techniques: Work with a speech therapist or occupational therapist who can teach the child specific swallowing techniques to manage dysphagia more effectively.

Speech Therapy: Regular sessions with a speech-language pathologist experienced in dysphagia can be beneficial. They can provide exercises and strategies tailored to the child's needs.

Medication Management: If the dysphagia is related to low muscle tone and there are medications that the child is taking to manage PWS symptoms, proper timing and administration of medication might improve their swallowing. I conduct constant exercises with our son and we go for walks daily to help him build muscle and strength. As previously mentioned, every drink I give him comes with a straw, to help him build strength with swallowing. We also do simple head and neck exercises, such as chin tucks or chin raises, neck stretches as this helps further. Constant hydration while eating also works as this keeps the throat moist and more functional. However, your speech-language pathologist can help you further in this space so it is best you speak to them.

As we approach the age of three, we are reaching a critical juncture. While the road ahead may become more challenging, it remains manageable with thoughtful decision-making. By this stage, you would have become acquainted with the PWS clinical medical team and are likely to have become part of the PWS clinic at your hospital, receiving invaluable guidance from the multidisciplinary team. The pivotal concept to grasp is 'management'. Every aspect of the PWS child's life requires meticulous management, far beyond what is typically encountered with a neurotypical child.

The journey of parenthood is akin to stepping into a world of magic and wonder, where the extraordinary becomes our reality. As I held my child, Aston-Martin, in my arms, I felt as though we had embarked on a quest akin to those in the tales of Hogwarts and the wizarding world. Little did I know that our path would take an unexpected turn, leading us into the heart of a rare and enigmatic condition — Prader-Willi Syndrome. It was as if we had stumbled upon a hidden chamber, revealing a world of challenges and unique magic.

With the diagnosis came a flood of emotions, from shock to determination, as we prepared to face this mysterious syndrome head-on. Thus began our adventure, armed with love, resilience, and a touch of wizarding wonder, ready to unlock the secrets of raising a child with extraordinary needs.

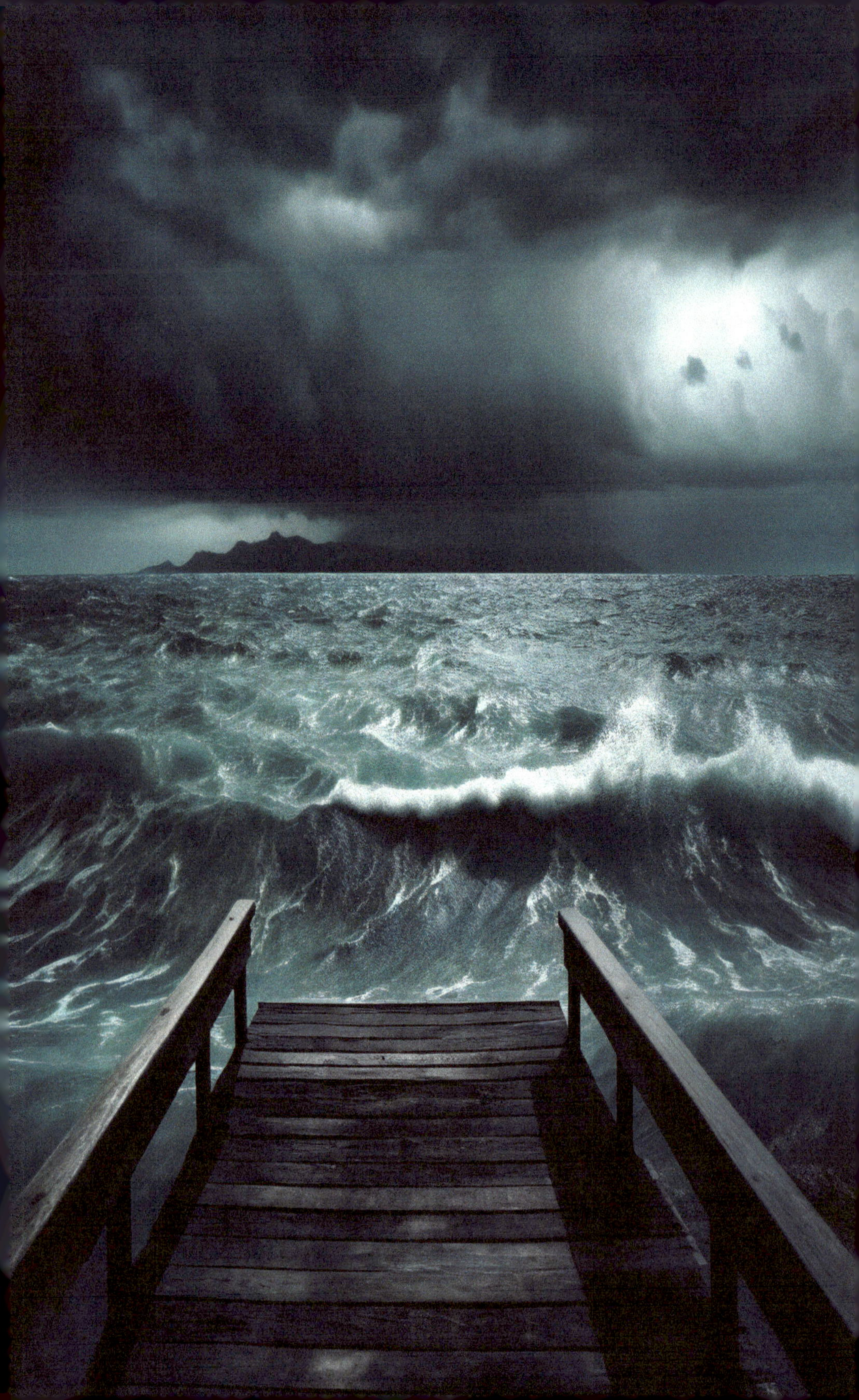

Chapter 6

The Awakening - Age Three

The early morning light filtered through the curtains, casting a soft glow over Aston-Martin's room, reminiscent of the first rays of dawn over the *enchanted Hogwarts grounds*. He lay quietly, his chest rising and falling with the steady rhythm of sleep. Yet even in these peaceful moments, his parents remained vigilant, much like the ever-watchful eyes of the castle's protective *spells*. They knew that the day ahead would be filled with the unique challenges that came with raising a child with Prader-Willi Syndrome.

It wasn't just the insatiable hunger that they had to manage; it was the myriad other symptoms that seemed to manifest in new ways each day. Aston-Martin's development was not like that of other children his age. His muscle tone was poor, and his movements lacked the fluidity and coordination of his peers. Speech therapy sessions had become a regular part of their weekly routine, as they worked diligently to help him overcome his language delays, much like a *young wizard* practising incantations for the first time.

As parents we often found ourselves being caught between the joy of witnessing our son's milestones and the fear of the health complications that lurked in the background. I remembered the first time Aston-Martin managed to string together a sentence. It was a moment of pure elation, quickly followed by the sobering reminder that his progress would always be shadowed by the realities of PWS, as if a *boggart* lurked in the shadows, ready to transform into their deepest fears.

As the day progressed, we navigated our carefully structured routine. Meals were planned with precision, portion sizes were measured, and snacks were kept out of sight. I had installed locks on the pantry and the refrigerator, a necessary precaution to prevent Aston-Martin from succumbing to his insatiable appetite, much like the protective enchantments around the *Philosopher's Stone*.

Despite our best efforts, there were moments when Aston-Martin's determination to find food led to heart-wrenching tantrums. We would hold him close, whispering words of comfort as he cried, his small hands reaching out for something, anything, to satisfy the hunger that never seemed to abate. It was in these moments that I felt the weight of my son's condition most acutely, a constant companion to the love I carried for him, as pervasive as the presence of magic in a *wizard's life*.

My dedication to maintaining a safe environment extended beyond the kitchen. Locking as much as I could, which was deemed necessary to prevent him from ever attempting to consume items, some of which were not even for human consumption. The locks on the fridge were temporarily in place, it would hold him off till at least four years of age, when his strength would increase. This now became a twenty-four-seven child.

I had learned to recognise the signs when Aston-Martin was about to engage in skin picking, a common behaviour in individuals with PWS. Distracting him became an art form, one that involved a delicate balance of attention and redirection, akin to the subtle art of potion-making, where each ingredient had to be added at just the right moment.

As I watched over Aston-Martin, I noticed moments when he seemed to retreat into a world of his own. It was as if he had found a secret passage in his mind, one that led to a place where the rest of the world couldn't follow. During these episodes, his eyes would fixate on a point in the distance, his gaze as still as the surface of the Black Lake on a windless night. He would be motionless, his little body frozen in time for more than 20 seconds.

At first, I thought these were moments of deep contemplation, akin to a *young wizard* lost in thought over an intricate spell. But as these episodes became more frequent, a niggling worry began to settle in my heart, whispering that this was something more than mere daydreaming.

It was during a routine visit to our *Healer*, a term I fondly used for their paediatrician, that I mentioned these peculiar *spells*. The *Healer* listened intently, her expression growing more serious with each detail I provided. She explained that while it was rarely mentioned in the clinical descriptions of PWS, seizures seemed to occur more frequently in those with the condition than in the general population. For Aston-Martin, she believed these were Absent Seizures.

The news hit me with the weight of a *Gringotts vault door*. Seizures were not a challenge I had prepared for, and the thought of my son experiencing them filled me with a sense of dread that was all too real. It was a reminder that PWS was a complex spell book, with pages that were sometimes difficult to read and understand, where indeed you would need to summon *Albus Dumbledore*.

Yet, with this new knowledge came a renewed sense of determination. I became ever more watchful, learning to recognize the signs of these seizures. We adapted our routine to ensure Aston-Martin's safety during these moments, creating a protective bubble around him much like the protective charms used in the wizarding world.

We consulted with specialists, delving deeper into the mysteries of PWS and how it intertwined with Aston-Martin's overall health for the mere fact he was only three years old and already showing intriguing characteristics. I was taught how to respond to these seizures, to gently guide my son back when the absent spell lifted. With each episode, we were there, a constant presence to anchor him in reality, to let him know he wasn't alone in whatever far-off land he visited.

In the quiet of the night, when the world seemed to hold its breath and the stars shone like tiny beacons of hope, I would sometimes allow myself to imagine that during these absent spells, Aston-Martin was visiting a place as magical as the wizarding world itself. A place where he could roam freely, unencumbered by the earthly limitations of PWS.

As I continued to face each day with courage, I found comfort in the thought that, much like the students of *Hogwarts* who faced their own trials, my family/friends too were learning, growing, and finding strength they never knew they had. And in this journey, the love we shared was the most powerful magic of all, a force that transcended the challenges and lit up the darkness with hope.

In the evenings, when Aston-Martin finally settled down to sleep, I would take a moment to breathe. I would sit, often in silence, reflecting on the day's successes and setbacks. I shared a bond with my other-self that was forged in the fires of adversity, a partnership that was as much about supporting my son as it was about supporting each other, not unlike the unbreakable friendships formed within the walls of *Hogwarts*.

I watched Aston-Martin with a mixture of fascination and concern as he engaged in one of his favourite activities—playing with water. His fascination seemed to border on an enchantment, reminiscent of the way a *young wizard* might be spellbound by their first successful levitation charm. He would take his drink bottle, his face alight with focus and delight, and he would fill it to the brim only to watch each drop cascade into a cup below. The sound of the water droplets, like a gentle pitter-patter of rain on the roof of *Hagrid's hut*, seemed to captivate him entirely.

When the skies above our home grew heavy with clouds, Aston-Martin would rush to find his umbrella, his eyes sparkling with anticipation. He would step out into the rain, standing still as a statue, simply listening to the symphony of raindrops. He could sit for what seemed like hours, lost in the rhythm of the water, as if it were a soothing incantation whispered by nature itself.

But it was his ritual with the cups that truly intrigued me. Aston-Martin would fill them up, then empty them out, only to begin the process anew. This repetitive action, a clear manifestation of his obsessive-compulsive tendencies, was both mesmerizing and a bit worrying. His relentless focus on the task was akin to a potion master absorbed in the perfect brewing of a complex concoction.

This particular fascination with water, however, was more than a simple childhood pastime; it was a part of the intricate tapestry of behaviours associated with Angelman Syndrome and not Prader-Willi Syndrome. The repetitive filling and emptying of cups, a soothing ritual, provided him with a sense of control, a way to make sense of his world. It was a behaviour that needed careful monitoring, ensuring it remained safe and did not interfere with his daily life.

As his parent, I took note of these moments, understanding that they were as much a part of Aston-Martin as his infectious laughter and his insatiable curiosity. I made sure to create a safe environment for him to indulge in his love for water, while also setting gentle boundaries to prevent any risks that could stem from his obsession.

In the tapestry of Aston-Martin's life, each thread — his love for the sound of rain, his fascination with the flow of water, his absent seizures, his challenges with food — was woven together to create a picture that was uniquely his own. It was a picture that required patience, love, and understanding to appreciate fully. And as his parent, I dedicated myself to providing him with all the support he needed to thrive, ensuring that his journey through life, though different, was as magical and filled with wonder as any tale from the world of *Harry Potter*.

I observed Aston-Martin's movements each day, noting the way he navigated the world with a unique determination. His coordination issues were evident; movements that came easily to other children required from him an effort as strenuous as a *young wizard* attempting to cast a spell for the very first time. Mobility, coordination, and strength difficulties were constant adversaries in his daily adventures, yet Aston-Martin faced them with the tenacity of a *Gryffindor*.

His gait was sometimes unsteady, his steps unsure, as if he were trying to walk across a moving staircase at *Hogwarts*. Each step required concentration, and I marvelled at his resolve not to let these challenges deter him from exploring his surroundings with the same enthusiasm as any other child. When Aston-Martin stumbled, I was there to offer a steadying hand, just as a professor might guide a student through a particularly difficult lesson.

Hand flapping was another behaviour I noticed, one more commonly associated with Angelman Syndrome than PWS. Aston-Martin would flap his hands when he was excited or anxious, a physical expression of his inner emotions. It was as though he had an inner energy that needed to be released, much like the sparks that fly from a wand when a spell is cast with particular fervour.

Delayed toilet training was yet another hurdle we faced together. Like a young wizard patiently practising the intricacies of potion-making, I patiently supported Aston-Martin through the process, understanding that for him, mastering this skill would take more time and patience. We celebrated the small victories, knowing that each step forward was a triumph over the challenges that PWS presented.

Through it all, I remained a vigilant guardian, a guide to help him navigate the complexities of his condition. I was there to celebrate his progress, to support him through setbacks, and to provide the love and encouragement he needed to continue growing and learning at his own pace.

In the grand scheme of things, these challenges were but one aspect of Aston-Martin's journey. They did not define him but rather shaped the way we, as a family, approached each day. We adapted, we learned, and we found joy in the small moments that others might take for granted. Our lives, much like the ever-changing halls of *Hogwarts*, were filled with unexpected twists and turns, but the love and magic we shared gave us the strength to face them together.

As Aston-Martin grew, so did the complexity of his needs. I sought out support groups and connected with other families who understood the unique journey of raising a child with PWS. They shared stories, exchanged tips, and found solace in the knowledge that they were not alone, creating a community as strong as *Dumbledore's* Army, united in their cause.

Through it all, Aston-Martin's spirit remained unbroken. His laughter was infectious, and his curiosity about the world around him was a constant source of delight. He loved to listen to music and would sway gently to the rhythms, a reminder that joy could be found even amidst the challenges, much like the wonder of discovering one's own patronus amid the darkness.

As the chapter of "The Awakening" came to a close, it was clear that the journey ahead for Aston-Martin and us, his family, would be one of continuous learning and adaptation. But it was also a journey filled with love, resilience, and the unspoken understanding that every moment, no matter how difficult, was precious, echoing the enduring magic found in the heart of every true friendship and family bond.

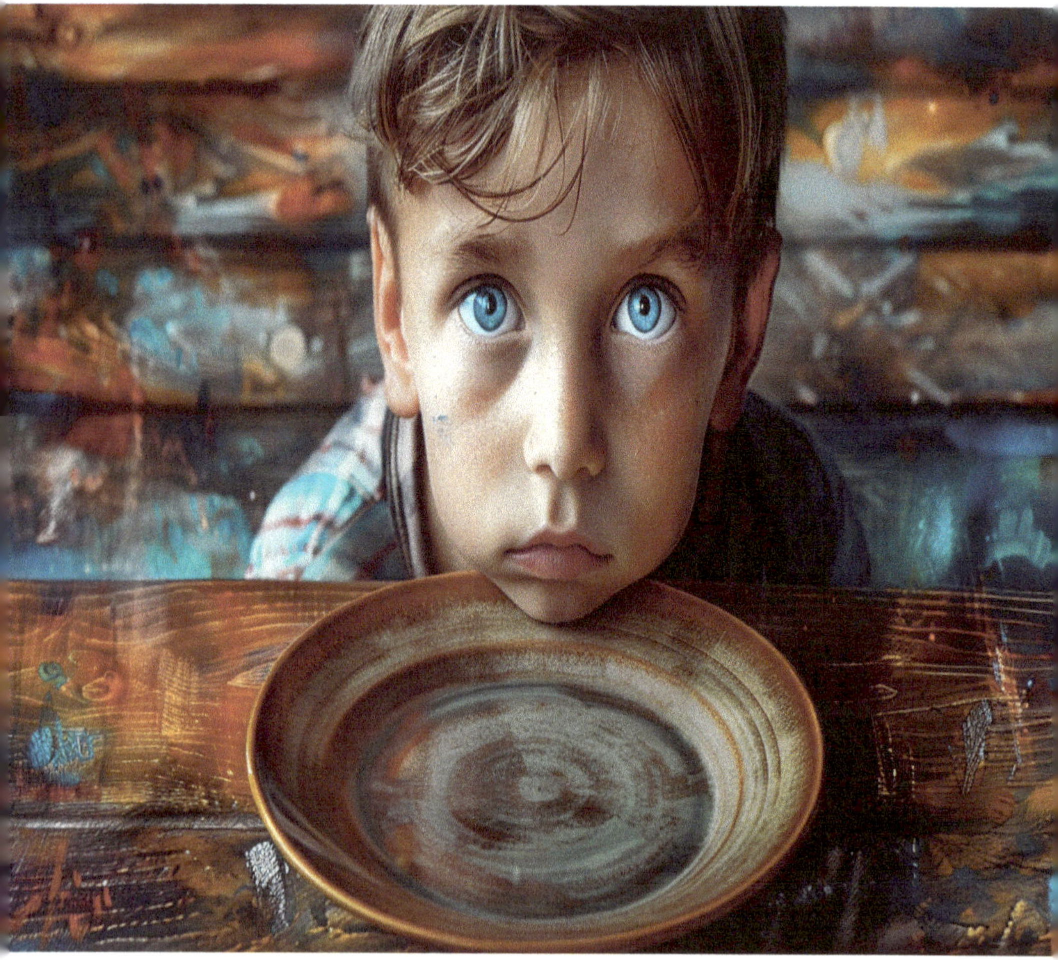

CHAPTER 7

The Dark Waters of Hunger - Age Four

I watched Aston-Martin with a heart that felt both heavy and hopeful. At four years old, his experience with hunger increased — until it was unlike anything most people could comprehend. It was as though he stood on the edge of a vast and dark lake, the waters of hunger stretching endlessly before him, never able to be fully crossed. His stomach seemed a bottomless pit, a constant echo of emptiness that no amount of food could silence.

This relentless hunger was a *Dementor* that haunted every moment of our daily lives, casting a shadow over Aston-Martin's otherwise bright and curious spirit. It was a force so palpable, as if the very air around us was thick with the weight of his constant need. His bright eyes, usually so full of wonder and mischief, would dim with the onset of this insatiable hunger, and I could see the struggle within him as he tried to articulate a hunger that words could not fully capture.

He was like a *young wizard* ensnared by an invisible force, his internal battle a silent scream for something as simple and as complicated as satiety. His small frame seemed to be under a spell, one that no incantation could break, no potion could cure. I watched as frustration built within him, his limited vocabulary unable to bridge the gap between his experience and my understanding. His emotions would swell like a storm over the Forbidden Forest, fierce and wild, until they broke forth in cries and screams that cut through me sharper than any *Sectumsempra curse*.

The depth of Aston-Martin's need was a chasm that seemed impossible to fill. He would reach for me, his hands grasping, his eyes pleading for relief from the relentless pull of hunger that gnawed at him. It was a cruel trick that his own body played on him, a never-ending charm of hunger cast by the very genes that made him who he was. I felt a profound helplessness, watching him grapple with a feeling that should have been within my power to alleviate, yet remained stubbornly beyond my reach.

In those moments, our home became a fortress, the kitchen a chamber of secrets that held the key to his temporary peace. The padlock on the fridge served as a necessary barrier, one that safeguarded him from the harm of his own unyielding desires. Yet, the sight of it was a constant reminder of the peculiar and painful reality we faced — a reality where the act of eating, so natural to most, was a complex ritual laden with danger for my son.

As the *Dementor* of hunger loomed over us, threatening to suck away the joy from our lives, I became more determined to find a way to cast a *Patronus* that could shield Aston-Martin from its effects. I sought out the wisdom of *healers* and fellow caregivers, arming myself with knowledge as one might arm themselves with spells and charms. We experimented with schedules and portion sizes, with textures and tastes, trying to find the combination that would provide the most comfort without exacerbating his condition.

We celebrated the good days when Aston-Martin would find a momentary distraction in his toys, his books, or the gentle touch of our family dog — a creature as loyal and protective as any *Hippogriff*. His laughter on those days was like a light in the darkness, a reminder of the love and happiness that still flourished in spite of the challenges we faced.

But the bad days were tough. There were times when no amount of distraction or comfort could ease the grip of hunger that held Aston-Martin in its clutches. On those days, I would hold him close, whispering words of comfort as if they were protective spells, hoping to offer him some solace until the feeling passed. I learned to recognise the subtle signs of his escalating anxiety, to intervene with a hug or a soothing word before the full force of his emotions could take hold.

It was during these times that I found my resolve tested, my own emotions a whirlwind of fear, sadness, and fierce protectiveness. Yet, it was also in these moments that I discovered the depth of my strength and the unbreakable bond that connected me to my son. Aston-Martin needed me to be his rock, his safe harbour in the midst of the storm, and I would not falter.

The journey was arduous, a path fraught with obstacles that seemed as insurmountable as the walls of *Azkaban*. But like any great saga, it was filled with moments of triumph and pure love that outshone the darkest of times. I knew that, together, we would continue to face each day with courage, weaving our *Patronus charms* into the fabric of our lives, creating a tapestry that told the story of a boy who could smile in the face of his *dementor*, and a family whose love was the most powerful magic of all.

Attempts to breach the defences of the padlocked fridge were frequent. Aston-Martin's small hands would grapple with the lock, his determination clashing with the cold, unyielding metal that kept him from his quest for sustenance. With each failed attempt, his cries and screams would fill the air, a raw expression of the battle he fought against his own body's unending demands.

In an effort to soothe his distress, we introduced a feedback toy — a small beacon of distraction amidst the turbulent waters. It vibrated, sang, and played melodies that seemed to enchant Aston-Martin, drawing his attention away from the call of hunger. The toy became a temporary port in the storm, a place where he could anchor his focus and find a moment's peace.

Yet the underlying current of hunger was ever-present, an adversary that required more than distractions to quell. We needed to be innovative and ever-watchful, crafting a strategy that balanced his nutritional needs with the importance of his emotional well-being. Each meal was planned with care, a delicate potion of necessary nutrients and the magic of comfort.

As we navigated further through the complexities of Aston-Martin's condition, we found ourselves facing a new set of challenges that I likened to dealing with the potions department — akin to the notorious *Slytherin house*, where things were not always as they seemed. To Aston-Martin, the colourful labels and intriguing shapes of household cleaning products were not warnings but invitations. In his eyes, the floor cleaner with its bright hue could easily be mistaken for a sweet cordial, and the aerosol of fly spray seemed as harmless as a can of deodorant.

Misidentification

It was a dangerous game of misidentification, one that led us on more than one occasion to the stark, white walls of *St Mungo's Hospital for Magical Maladies and Injuries*. My heart sank the day Aston-Martin suffered chemical burns because he had assumed the floor cleaner was a suitable body wash. The sight of his delicate skin, red and angry from the harsh chemicals, was a stark reminder of the vigilance his world required. It was a painful lesson that our home was filled with potions that could harm as much as heal, and that our little *wizard's* curiosity could lead to dire consequences.

From then on, I knew that we had to transform our home into a place of safety, a stronghold against the potential poisons that lurked within. Every cupboard and shelf became a subject of scrutiny. I moved all accessible items from bottom to top, out of the reach of inquisitive hands. The locks we installed were not just physical barriers but charms of protection, meant to shield Aston-Martin from the allure of these forbidden bottles.

The task was daunting, as if I were rearranging the entire contents of *Weasley's Wizard Wheezes* to ensure that only the harmless joke products were within reach of a child. Each item had to be considered for its potential risk, each placement strategic. It was a process that required the foresight of a chess master, anticipating moves and countermoves in an ongoing battle for safety.

In our quest to prevent more 'booms' from mixing these dangerous 'potions,' our home began to resemble a puzzle, each piece meticulously placed to create a cohesive picture of security. I labelled cabinets with clear warnings and educated Aston-Martin on the dangers as best I could, hoping that the information would seep in and provide an additional layer of defence against his innate curiosity.

Despite these precautions, I knew that supervision was the key. Like a hawk-eyed professor overseeing a room full of *young witches and wizards brewing Polyjuice Potion*, I kept a watchful eye on Aston-Martin. I created a schedule that allowed for structured activities and limited the opportunities for him to seek out the forbidden items that so intrigued him.

The world through Aston-Martin's eyes was one of wonder and exploration, where every object held the potential for discovery. It was a trait I cherished, even as I worked to channel it into safer avenues. We introduced new 'potions' in the form of sensory play — water mixed with food colouring, safe-to-touch slime, and doughs that allowed him to experiment and mix to his heart's content without risk of harm.

Chapter 7.1

Breaking the Cycle - Age Four

Our frequent visits to the St Mungo's Hospital for Magical Maladies and Injuries became a tapestry woven into the fabric of our lives, each thread a different shade of worry and urgency. The emergency room, with its beeping monitors and the antiseptic smell, became an all-too-familiar setting. The cause was often a rash that bloomed across Aston-Martin's skin, a fiery red map that charted an invisible territory of pain. Initially, we would fear he had ingested something harmful, but it would turn out that he had used cleaning products in an attempt to wash himself. His body, sensitive and reactive, would flare up in protest, and there I would be, his father, heart pounding in my chest as I raced to the hospital, fearing that my son was about to dissolve like sugar in tea.

The irony of the situation was not lost on me. The hospital, a place of healing, also became a place of temptation. Its corridors were lined with the very things that we kept under lock and key at home. Ice cream, drinks, sandwiches, cookies — these were the treats that the doctors and nurses would offer as a form of currency to coax Aston-Martin into compliance. It was a practical solution to the immediate problem; the promise of a treat would allow them to draw blood, administer medication, or collect a urine sample. And Aston-Martin, with his insatiable hunger, never once declined.

The staff, with their well-meaning intentions, didn't fully understand the complexity of the situation. Each treat was a reinforcement of an association that was slowly taking root in Aston-Martin's mind: the hospital was a place where the forbidden became accessible. He was taking mental notes, and soon, he began to see the hospital as a destination for indulgence rather than a place for treatment.

Aston-Martin's pain tolerance, a trait common in individuals with Prader-Willi Syndrome, added another layer of complexity. His cries of pain were not to be taken lightly, as they signified a level of discomfort that would incapacitate the average person. So, when he would scream or cry, indicating that something was amiss, we would rush him to the hospital, fearing the worst, only to find that the promise of treats would miraculously alleviate his symptoms.

It was a cunning and oddly endearing aspect of his personality, this desire to find a way to the things he craved. But as he grew older, it developed into a pattern that was both dangerous and heartbreaking. He learned that self-inflicted harm could be a ticket to the treats he coveted, and so the cycle began. A minor bump could transform into a dramatic performance, and off we would go, sirens blaring in my mind, to the land of ice cream and custard.

It wasn't until I had a *Rubeus Hagrid* moment, that the pieces of the puzzles started to fall into place for me. One particularly harrowing episode saw us in the hospital once more, with Aston-Martin in apparent agony from stomach pain and a headache. The staff, following their established protocol, offered him the usual array of treats, and like magic, his ailments seemed to vanish. He could walk, sit up, and his demeanour brightened considerably. Aston-Martin's communication was still limited, but the transformation was stark.

Once we returned home, he was back to his usual self, rummaging through cupboards with a relentless drive to find something to eat. It was then that I realised the depth of the association he had formed and the lengths he would go to satisfy his hunger. The hospital was no longer just a place of healing for him; it was a place where the rules of home did not apply.

I knew then that we needed to break this cycle. I began to communicate more with the hospital staff, explaining the nuances of Prader-Willi Syndrome and the importance of not using food as a reward. Together, we developed new strategies for managing his care during hospital visits, strategies that did not involve the treats that had become such a powerful motivator for him.

The journey was far from over, and the learning curve was steep. Each day brought new challenges, but also new insights into the complex world of my son. I learned to navigate the delicate balance between meeting his needs and managing his condition, all the while loving him for the unique and wonderful person he was. Our bond, tested and forged in the fires of these experiences, became unbreakable. And I held onto the hope that with patience, understanding, and unwavering love, we would find our way through the maze of Prader-Willi Syndrome, one step at a time.

As the days turned into weeks, and weeks into months, the incidents became fewer. The combination of physical safeguards, constant vigilance, and redirection towards safe activities began to take effect. Aston-Martin learned, in his own way, which items were not to be touched, and the locks on the cabinets remained undisturbed.

Yet even with the most meticulous of systems in place, the worry never fully dissipated. It lingered in the background, a constant reminder that the world was not as benign as it might seem. But in the face of this reality, our family's resilience grew. We adapted, we learned, and we found strength in the knowledge that each day we overcame these trials was a victory in itself.

Our home had become the prison of Azkaban fortress, not just of locks and labels, but of love and learning. And though the journey was fraught with challenges, it was also filled with growth and the kind of love that could only be forged in the fires of adversity. In the end, I knew that the greatest protection I could offer Aston-Martin was not just the safety of our home, but the sanctuary of our family's embrace, where he would always be loved, always be safe, and always be free to explore the magic of his world, within the bounds of our careful guardianship.

At the tender age of four and a half, Aston-Martin's innocent and trusting nature revealed itself in a way that was both endearing and terrifying. I observed with a mix of emotions as he would reach out his small hand to clasp that of a stranger, his gesture as natural to him as breathing. To onlookers, the sight was heartwarming — a symbol of the inherent trust children have in the world around them. But the implications of this behaviour were anything but warm or heartening. It was a vulnerability that we, as his parents, could not afford to overlook.

His indiscriminate willingness to hold hands with anyone presented a stark contrast to the instinctive caution most children his age displayed. Where another four-year-old might recognise their parents' faces and voices with certainty, Aston-Martin did not. He seemed to lack the concept of 'stranger danger' entirely. While he sat in his stroller, his little hand would snake out in search of another's, and if a passerby, taken by his sweet demeanour, accepted it, his face would light up with joy. He would laugh and engage with them as if they were his closest kin.

This was not a simple phase or a harmless quirk. Over the year, this trait became deeply ingrained, and the potential consequences grew more severe. The thought of him placing his trust so readily in a stranger filled me with dread. The very idea that he might one day be led away by someone he mistook for a parent was the stuff of nightmares. It was a life-or-death situation, a reality check that our son's perception of the world differed vastly from the norm.

In Aston-Martin's case, there was no fear, no hesitation. His world was one without the boundaries that fear imposes, without the intuitive suspicion that keeps most children safe. It was a beautiful innocence, but one that could not be left unguarded. We had to teach him, somehow, to discern friend from foe, to understand that not every hand extended towards him was safe to take.

We began to implement strategies to help him learn. We practised at home, role-playing scenarios where he had to look for us before accepting anyone else's hand. We used social stories and visual cues to reinforce the lesson that he had one mum and one dad, and that it was only safe to go with people he recognised and trusted. We made a game of it, trying to instil the lesson in a way that was engaging for him, yet the gravity of the situation was never far from my mind.

In public, we became ever more vigilant. Our eyes were constantly scanning the environment, our hands always within reach of his. We spoke to him in clear and simple terms, reminding him to stay close, to check with us before interacting with others. We attached colourful wristbands with our contact information to his wrists, a small measure of security in the vast and unpredictable sea of people.

The stroller became a chariot of sorts, a vehicle through which we could navigate the crowds while keeping him safely contained. But as he grew, so too did his reach, and the stroller could not be a permanent solution. We had to trust in our efforts, in the lessons we repeated daily, and in the small increments of understanding we saw in him.

It was an ongoing battle against a world that could not be made entirely safe, against a condition that stripped away the natural barriers most of us take for granted. But it was a battle we approached with determination, with the knowledge that every small victory was a step towards his safety.

As we moved through this journey, I came to realise that the trust Aston-Martin placed in the world was a reflection of the trust he placed in us, his parents. It was our job to be worthy of that trust, to protect him until he could learn to protect himself. And though the path was fraught with anxiety and uncertainty, it was also filled with moments that reminded me of the beauty of his trust — the way he would snuggle into my arms, certain of his sanctuary, the way his laughter could light up the darkest of days.

We would teach him caution, yes, but I hoped that the world would not teach it to him too harshly. I hoped that as he learned to navigate the complexities of life, he would retain some of that beautiful trust, that it would be tempered but not extinguished, and that it would serve not as a weakness but as a testament to the boundless capacity for love that lived within him.

Aston-Martin's journey through this dark water was a testament to the power of resilience, both his and ours. The limitations imposed by his age and the barriers to communication made the struggle all the more poignant. It was a dance between the need to protect him and the need to empower him, to help him find his voice in expressing his hunger without being overwhelmed by it.

Understanding became our wand, empathy our spell. We learned to read the silent language of his needs, to anticipate the rise and fall of his hunger like the ebb and flow of the tide. We became the guardians of his wellbeing, the keepers of the calm in the midst of his storm.

As Aston-Martin's story unfolded, it was clear that the journey through the dark waters of hunger was not one we could navigate alone. It required the support of a community, the charms club, the potions club and the wisdom of those who had charted these waters before us, and the unspoken bond of a family united in love and purpose.

And through it all, I held onto the belief that with each day, with each challenge we overcame, we were not just moving through these dark waters but transforming them, drop by drop, into a wellspring of strength and understanding that would nourish Aston-Martin's soul just as much as any meal could nourish his body.

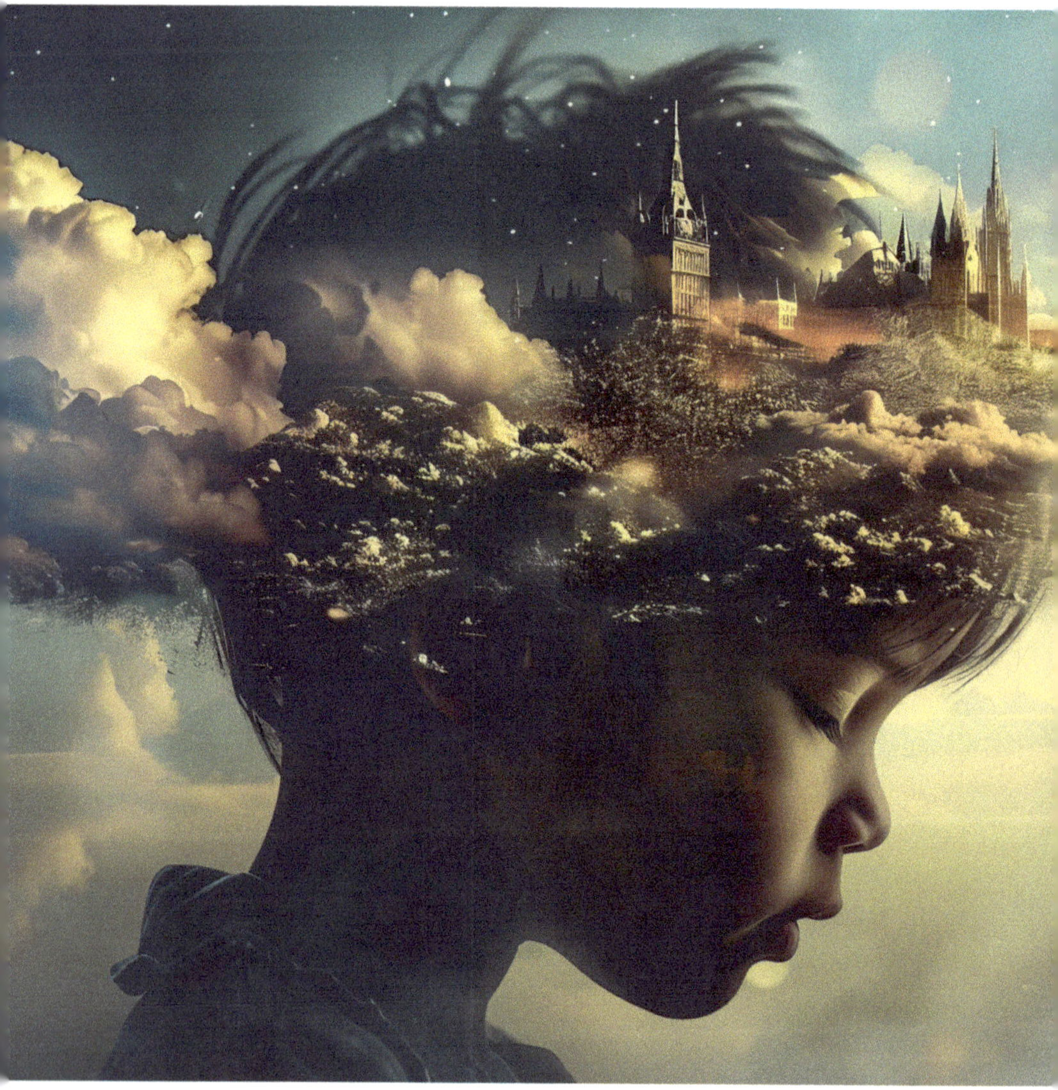

Chapter 8

The Discovery - Age Five

The day was bright with possibility, much like walking into the Great Hall at Hogwarts for the first time, the ceiling reflecting the sky's azure expanse and the tables laden with expectation. It was a day of discovery, a day when new doors would open for Aston-Martin, my bright and curious five-year-old boy whose spirit was as uncontainable as a Cornish pixie.

My wife, a woman of unwavering determination and the kind of love that could move mountains, was on a mission. She sought a childcare centre that would embrace Aston-Martin not just as a child, but as a little wizard with his own set of spells and enchantments. Our previous attempts had been disheartening, to say the least. One centre, cloaked in ignorance like a Dementor in its dark shroud, had turned us away, their prejudice a cold wind that bit at our heels as we left.

But she persevered, her wand of hope casting light in the shadows until we found a place that seemed to have been touched by the warmth of a Patronus. This new childcare centre radiated acceptance and understanding, promising to prioritise the safety and wellbeing of every child within its walls.

The director, a kind-hearted witch with a twinkle in her eye that reminded me of Professor McGonagall, assured us that Aston-Martin would be cared for as one of their own. She spoke of the centre's inclusive philosophy, where every child's uniqueness was celebrated, and I saw the relief wash over my wife's face like the calming effect of a well-brewed Draught of Peace.

Aston-Martin, with the wide-eyed wonder of a young wizard exploring Diagon Alley for the first time, ventured into the centre. His laughter echoed through the brightly coloured halls as he discovered toys and books that sparked his imagination. He was drawn to an obstacle course, a miniature version of a *Quidditch pitch*, complete with hoops and soft broomsticks.

But as he climbed atop a cushioned platform, misfortune struck like a rogue Bludger, and he fell. My wife, ever the vigilant guardian, was at his side in an instant, her heart pounding like the wings of a *Hippogriff* in flight. She cradled him, checking for injuries as she reiterated the importance of a one-to-one ratio for his care, much like *Harry Potter* needed the close companionship of *Ron* and *Hermione*.

Her voice was firm yet kind as she explained the nuances of Prader-Willi Syndrome to the staff, who listened with a mix of concern and fascination. She spoke of the constant vigilance required, the monitoring of food intake, and the need for physical security. It was clear that Aston-Martin could not simply be left to navigate the world alone; he needed a *Hagrid* to his *Harry*, a guide and protector who understood the depth of his condition.

She had come prepared, armed with pamphlets and recommendations for allied health support, her own version of *Hermione's* beaded bag, filled with solutions and spells for every occasion. The childcare centre, however, hesitated, as if the idea of accommodating such needs was as complex as the *Triwizard Tournament*. They worried about the extra resources required, the potential disruptions to their established routine, and the challenge of integrating such support into their environment.

The encounter was a stark reminder of the barriers that families like ours often face. The wizarding world was not always kind to those who were different, and the *Muggle* world, it seemed, was no different. We were the parents of a child who needed more than the standard incantations and charms. Our son required a level of care that went beyond the basic *Expecto Patronum*; he needed a tailored spell-book, a custom wand crafted to fit his hand alone.

But we would not be deterred. My wife, with the same resolve that had carried her through the halls of *St. Mungo's* and the corridors of countless specialists, would not accept defeat. She advocated for Aston-Martin with the eloquence of *Dumbledore*, the determination of *McGonagall*, and the resourcefulness of *Hermione*.

Our quest became one of education, of opening minds and hearts to the reality of our son's world. We sought understanding and empathy, allies in a world that could be as daunting as any Forbidden Forest. We worked tirelessly to build bridges, and to create a network of support that would allow Aston-Martin to thrive in this new environment.

The journey was long and filled with obstacles, much like the path to destroying *Horcruxes*. But we were steadfast. We held onto the belief that with patience, love, and a little magic, we could find a way to give Aston-Martin the care he deserved, to help him grow and learn in a place where he was seen not as a burden, but as a boy with boundless potential.

And so, the chapter of discovery continued each day a new page in the story of our little wizard. It was a tale of challenges and triumphs, of the love that shone like the brightest *Lumos* in the darkest of nights. We were his family, his guardians, his champions, and together, we would navigate the enchanting and complicated world that lay before us.

As I navigated the labyrinthine corridors of the Early Childhood Development Program (ECDP) at the special school, I couldn't help but feel like I was stepping into a world as complex and unfamiliar as the Department of Mysteries. Aston-Martin had been attending ECDP twice per week since he was four, a place designed to be a nurturing ground for young minds like his, where the magic of early education was tailored to the unique needs of each child.

Twice a week, we would embark on this journey together, with me at his side, much like a young wizard and their familiar. It was a partnership, a duet between parent and child, as we explored the realms of socialising, colour recognition, painting, and play. The goal was to establish a routine, a rhythm to our days that would provide Aston-Martin with the predictability and structure he so desperately needed.

His communication was akin to the secret language of *Parseltongue*, understood by few, and often misinterpreted by many. His verbal skills were limited to a symphony of sounds and the occasional word, most of which were related to his ceaseless hunger. It was a language I had come to understand, though it was foreign to my ears when I first heard it.

The ECDP environment was new to me, a place where the lines between the *Muggle world* and the *wizarding* one seemed to blur. I had no prior experience with special schools, and I entered with trepidation, half-expecting an owl to arrive with a letter of apology and a redirection to a mainstream school. I harboured a secret hope that perhaps they had misdiagnosed him, that my memories of my own primary school, filled with warmth and simplicity, would become his.

But the anticipated call never came. Instead, I found myself immersed in a classroom that was a patchwork of diversity, where each child had their own story, their own set of challenges woven into the very fabric of their being. As I looked around at the other children, with their wide array of genetic and chromosomal conditions, I felt a kinship with the other parents. I understood the sacrifices they had made, the lives put on pause, reshaped and remoulded to support the needs of their extraordinary children.

The reality of our situation was stark. Just like many of the parents there, I had exhausted all forms of leave from my job — annual, sick, and carer's. I had been a soldier once, but now I faced a different kind of battle, one that required a different kind of resilience. My savings, once earmarked for a house, became a lifeline in a sea of medical appointments and therapies.

The stress was colossal, a towering troll that I had to face with the same courage *Harry Potter* showed in the *dungeons of Hogwarts*. My military injuries, which I carried like invisible scars, were a constant reminder of the life I had once known. And now, faced with the realisation that maintaining a job was a near-impossible task, I grappled with the weight of our new reality.

Aston-Martin was a 24/7 child, his needs as constant as the stars in the night sky. The number of appointments was overwhelming, a relentless tide that no amount of annual leave could hope to contain.

My savings, once a beacon of hope for a future home, began to dwindle as I used them to navigate the treacherous waters of our daily life. It was not what they were intended for, but what is gold compared to the wellbeing of one's child?

In the wizarding world, one could conjure necessities with a flick of a wand, but in the harsh light of reality, no such magic existed. There were no Time-Turners to extend the hours of the day to accommodate the relentless schedule of appointments and care.

Yet, within the walls of ECDP, there was a different kind of magic at work — a magic born of compassion, understanding, and the shared experiences of families like ours. It was a place where Aston-Martin could flourish, where his unique way of being was not just accepted but celebrated.

As I watched him interact with his peers, engage in activities that sparked joy in his eyes, I knew that this was where he needed to be. The road ahead was fraught with uncertainty, but it was a path we would navigate together, with the love and determination that had seen us through thus far.

The journey was far from over, and the challenges we faced were daunting.

Kitchen nightmares

At age of five and a half, Aston-Martin's fascination with the kitchen became as evident as the enchantment of a well-cast *Lumos* spell in a darkened room. It was during my visits to the ECDP that an epiphany struck me like *Hagrid's* air biscuit (that's rudimentary English for fart) of a seasoned wizard. The toys that he was so fond of at school — pans, stoves, cups, forks, and spoons — were not just playthings, but tools of mimicry, shaping his actions at home.

The duality of this revelation was as clear as the dichotomy between good and evil in the wizarding world. It was good, a sign that he was learning, absorbing the routines and practices from school and replicating them in the comfort of our home. Yet, there was a darker side to this, much like the hidden dangers lurking within the *Forbidden Forest*. His association of the kitchen with food was growing stronger, and his attempts to engage with it became increasingly risky. The stove, a benign object at ECDP, turned into a source of peril in our *Muggle* kitchen as he tried to activate it, unaware of the real-world consequences.

When I intervened, it was as if I had cast a *Silencing Charm* on his playtime. Outbursts would follow — cries and yells that echoed the frustration of a young wizard unable to continue his magical experiments. These emotional spells were small at first, but like the growing power of a young sorcerer, they intensified with age.

Addressing his nutritional needs was akin to potion-making, a delicate balance of ingredients and measurements. Aston-Martin had his own unique naming conventions for various edibles, and 'muesli bar' became a term as familiar to us as 'Chocolate Frog' is to a *Hogwarts* student. Ensuring his health, I became as discerning as a witch or wizard selecting wand wood, purchasing only muesli bars that met the high standards of Australia's 'Star' system. With a threshold of no less than 3.5 stars, I made no exceptions, much like a potion master refuses to use subpar ingredients.

I transformed our kitchen into a place of culinary magic, where every item was as organic and wholesome as the produce from *Hagrid's garden*. This way, if Aston-Martin ever embarked on an unsupervised foraging expedition while I was momentarily absent, the foods he encountered would be as harmless as a *Flobberworm*. It was a strategy born of necessity; a protective enchantment woven into the very fabric of our daily lives.

The kitchen, once a simple room for preparing meals, had evolved into a place of learning and potential mishaps. I had to be ever-vigilant, like a member of the *Order of the Phoenix* on watch, ready to intervene should the need arise. My role was to guide and protect, to teach him the difference between the harmless play at ECDP and the very real dangers of our home environment.

Yet, in this challenge, there was also a spellbinding beauty. Watching Aston-Martin engage with the world around him, learning and growing despite the obstacles he faced, was a reminder of the extraordinary magic of the human spirit. Each day was a lesson, each interaction a chance to impart knowledge and understanding, much like a professor at *Hogwarts* guiding their students through the complexities of spell work and life.

The journey was fraught with trials, but like any good tale, it was the love and dedication that shone through the darkest moments. Aston-Martin's journey, with its unique blend of challenges and triumphs, was our own magical adventure—one that we would continue to navigate with the resilience of a *Gryffindor*, the intelligence of a *Ravenclaw*, the dedication of a *Hufflepuff*, and the ambition of a *Slytherin*. Together, we would conquer the challenges, celebrate the victories, and above all, ensure that the kitchen remained a place of nourishment and joy, rather than danger.

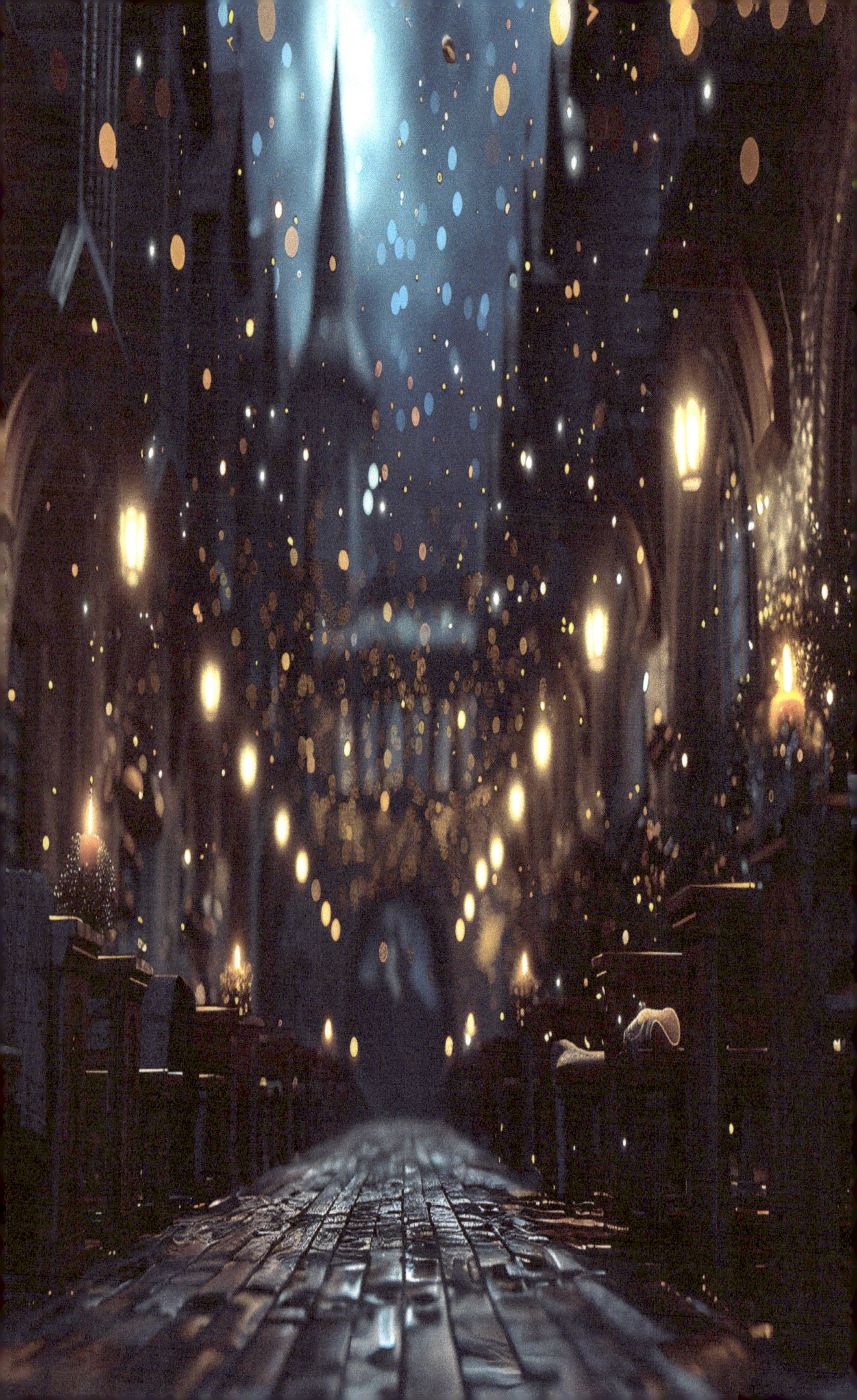

Chapter 9

The Mystoria School of Magic - Day One - Age Six

The morning sun cast a warm glow over the quaint little house where Aston-Martin, was about to embark on a remarkable journey. Today marked his first day in Year One at a special school, a day filled with anticipation and a flutter of anxiety that danced in his stomach like Cornish pixies.

Aston-Martin's parents, who had always been his most ardent supporters, bustled around him with a mix of pride and excitement. They adjusted his backpack, smoothed his hair, and shared reassuring smiles that seemed to say, "You're off to discover your own brand of magic, and we're right here with you." As they accompanied him to school, their hearts swelled with hope, eager to witness how their little boy would integrate into this new world and how he would cope with the adventures that lay ahead.

Stepping into the classroom at the *Mystoria School of Magic*, a place of learning and growth for children like Aston-Martin, was like entering a scene from a storybook. The room was a tapestry of colours, each hue more vibrant than the last, and it was filled to the brim with toys and activities designed to engage the curious minds of its young inhabitants. From enchanted puzzles that sang when completed to storybooks that whispered their tales, everything in the room was meticulously chosen to spark wonder and learning.

The support system was formidable, with one teacher and five teacher aids, each one a guardian of these young minds. They provided the personalised attention that each student required, becoming the gentle guides in a world that could sometimes feel as vast and mysterious as the Forbidden Forest.

Aston-Martin, with the wide-eyed innocence of a child stepping into *Diagon Alley* for the first time, moved from one toy to another, his concentration as fleeting as a snitch in flight. This hinted at his potential Attention-deficit/hyperactivity disorder ADHD, a condition that made the world a blur of excitement, too vast to be contained in a single moment.

In the corner of the room, a small tent stood like a sanctuary, its fabric walls a shield from the outside world. Here, children could retreat into their own private nook, a place of calm and security akin to the comforting embrace of an *Invisibility Cloak*. It was a reminder that even in a room full of magic and play, there was a space for solitude and peace when the world became too overwhelming.

The routine of the school day was a well-oiled machine, with transportation to and from school provided on a bus that seemed as magical as the Knight Bus itself, albeit without the breakneck speed. It eased the burden on families, allowing them to breathe a little easier, knowing their children were in safe hands as they journeyed to and from their place of learning.

As the day unfolded, Aston-Martin's initial apprehension melted away like chocolate frogs in the sun. He found joy in the simple acts of painting, building, and even in the routine of snack time, where he was learning to manage his PWS with the guidance of his attentive teachers. We, his parents watched, our hearts a mixture of relief and pride, as our son navigated his first day with the bravery of a young wizard facing his first spell.

The Mystoria School of Magic, nestled within the heart of a world that wasn't quite like the one you and I know, was a place where the extraordinary was nurtured with the same care as *Professor Sprout* tended to her magical plants. Within its enchanted walls, Aston-Martin, my son, was like a young wizard discovering his powers, his attention pulled in every direction by the allure of new discoveries. Each toy beckoned to him with the promise of a new spell to master, yet his ability to focus on any single enchantment was as fleeting as the flight of a *Golden Snitch*.

It was during these moments of frenetic activity that his teacher, a perceptive sorceress in her own right, observed Aston-Martin's pattern. She noted that his concentration was as easily broken as a *Protego* charm facing a powerful curse. This, she mused, could be the work of an unseen magical spell known as Attention-deficit/hyperactivity disorder (ADHD), which made the tasks at hand as slippery and elusive as trying to grasp a handful of *Gilly weed*.

Recognising that this spell required a special kind of countercharm, she recommended seeking the expertise of specialists from a renowned department, a place where the mysteries of the mind were unravelled with the same care as ancient runes. This fabled place was none other than the Department of Paediatric Wizardry, an institution where the medical magicians, or paediatricians as they are known in the *Muggle* world, delved into the complexities of conditions like ADHD with the precision of a wand carving intricate patterns into the air.

The Department of Paediatric Wizardry was not just a place of diagnosis and treatment; it was a sanctuary where the unique attributes of each young wizard and witch were understood and embraced. Here, the paediatricians, with their vast knowledge of magical maladies, worked tirelessly to ensure that every child could harness their own form of magic, regardless of the spells that may have been cast upon them.

Alongside the recommendation to consult with the Department of Paediatric Wizardry, she also suggested to us that Aston-Martin meet with a speech pathologist from the equally esteemed

Department of Linguistic Charms. This department was a marvel in itself, a place where words and sounds were woven together with the same care as *Madame Malkin* stitched wizarding robes. The speech pathologists within were akin to wandmakers, each word and syllable carefully crafted and tailored to the needs of the young minds they guided.

Aston-Martin's first encounter with his speech pathologist was as transformative as a first-year *Hogwarts* student's introduction to their house. The pathologist, with a twinkle in her eye that could rival that of *Dumbledore's*, greeted him warmly, inviting him into a world where language was not just a means of communication, but a gateway to a realm of possibility.

Under her guidance, Aston-Martin began to explore the cadence and rhythm of speech, each word a note in the symphony of language. The pathologist's room was filled with enchanted objects designed to aid in this quest — a mirror that would repeat words with perfect pronunciation, picture cards that came to life to illustrate their meaning, and a magical quill that would only write the correct form of words spoken aloud.

As days turned into weeks, Aston-Martin's progress was steady and sure. The once elusive concentration began to anchor itself more firmly with each session, much like a spell taking hold after several attempts. His ability to focus on a single task grew stronger, not unlike a young wizard mastering their first levitation charm.

The Department of Paediatric Wizardry and the Department of Linguistic Charms became integral parts of Aston-Martin's world. The specialists within these departments worked hand-in-hand with the *Mystoria School of Magic*, creating a support network as strong and as intricate as the spells woven into the tapestry of *Hogwarts* itself.

The journey was not without its challenges, of course. There were moments when the ADHD spell seemed to strengthen its grip, making each toy in the classroom as distracting as a room full of *bewitched bludgers*. Yet, with the unwavering support of his teachers, the expertise of the paediatric wizards, and the magic of speech therapy, Aston-Martin continued to grow and thrive.

We, ever-present and ever-supportive, watched with a mixture of awe and relief as our son navigated this enchanted world. We observed the once overwhelming kitchen become a place of order and learning, where Aston-Martin could safely experiment with the alchemy of cooking under their watchful eyes. We witnessed his speech blossoming like a rare flower, each new word a petal unfurling in the warmth of the sun.

The chapter closed on a positive note, with Aston-Martin's laughter ringing in the air, a melody more delightful than any song. My wife and I exchanged glances, a silent conversation passing between us that spoke volumes of our journey ahead — a journey filled with challenges, yes, but also brimming with the potential for growth, learning, and happiness. We knew that the *Mystoria School of Magic* would be a place where Aston-Martin could flourish, his unique traits nurtured and celebrated, and where every day would be a testament to the magic that exists in every child's heart.

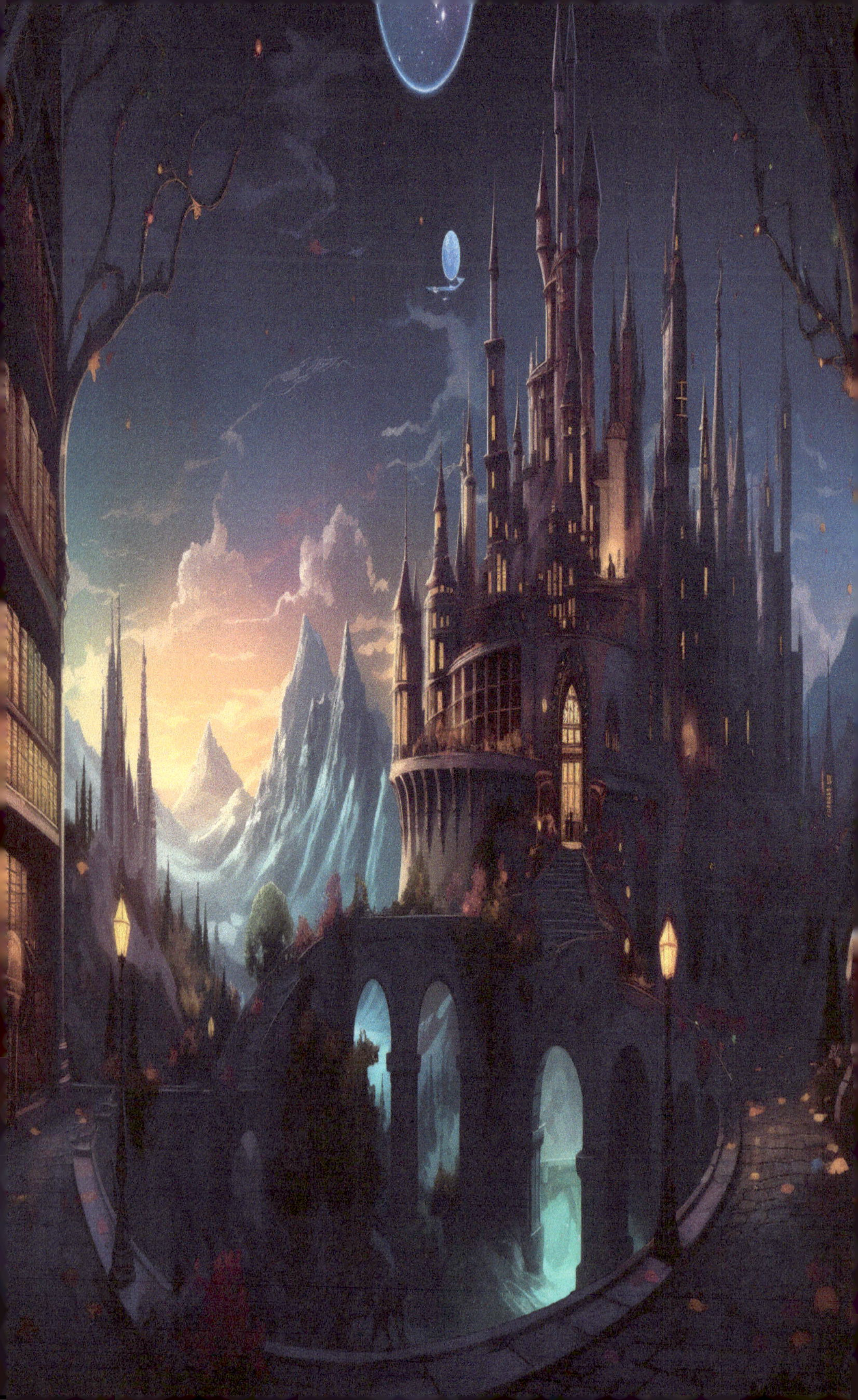

CHAPTER 10

The Department of Paediatric Wizardry, and the Department of Linguistic Charms - Age Six

The Mystoria School of Magic, the Department of Paediatric Wizardry, and the Department of Linguistic Charms — these were the pillars of Aston-Martin's world, the cornerstones of his development. Together, they formed a constellation of care that guided him through his formative years, ensuring that his unique magic was not just preserved, but allowed to shine as brightly as the most powerful Lumos spell.

As Aston-Martin's journey at the *Mystoria School of Magic* unfolded, his condition — much like a persistent *Niffler* — drove him to seek out food with an ever-increasing determination as he became older. His Prader-Willi Syndrome fuelled a relentless hunger, a craving for sustenance as powerful as the most potent of love potions. This urge led him to embark on late-night clandestine missions, tiptoeing through the shadows of our home with the stealth of an accomplished *Auror* on a covert operation, in search of the treasures hidden within the cupboards.

Despite the enchantments placed around the kitchen, designed to deter such quests — charms of sound that would alert me to the opening of doors, locks that required a touch of magic only I possessed — Aston-Martin's ingenuity knew no bounds. He was a young *Marauder* in his own right, his mind always searching for a way around the spells meant to protect him from his own insatiable appetite.

At school, his craftiness was no less evident. With the subtlety of an *Invisibility Cloak* draped over his intentions, he would watch his fellow young wizards and witches, awaiting the perfect moment to liberate a piece of fruit or a biscuit from their unsuspecting grasp. It wasn't malice that drove him, but a charm he couldn't break — a charm that made food seem as irresistible as the song of a *Veela*.

His talent for misdirection was as impressive as that of a professional *Quidditch Seeker* dodging *Bludgers*; he had an uncanny ability to hide food for later consumption. The classroom, a place of learning and wonder, also became a cache of secret stashes. Beneath a pile of spell books, behind a curtain of colourful beads, or within the hollow of a toy cauldron, he would conceal his contraband, ensuring that he had reserves should the need arise.

At home, too, he found nooks and crannies that even I, with all my vigilance, had overlooked. Behind the sofa cushions, within the cozy confines of his sock drawer, and in the shadowy space beneath his bed, he hid his treasures. He outsmarted us all — his teachers, his peers, and yes, even me, the grandaddy of them all. His strategies were as cunning and resourceful as those employed by the young heroes of the wizarding world in their battles against dark forces.

I couldn't help but admire his cleverness, even as I worried for his health. The enchantments around the house became more complex, the monitoring spells more intricate. I sought counsel from the specialists at the Department of Paediatric Wizardry, wizards and witches well-versed in the nuances of PWS. Together, we crafted a plan as meticulously as a potion master creates a *Polyjuice Potion*, aiming to manage Aston-Martin's condition without stifling his spirit.

The Department of Linguistic Charms also played a role in this delicate balance. His speech pathologist, a wise sorceress with a gentle voice, used her skills to help him express his needs and desires without resorting to secrecy. She employed enchanted tools that encouraged communication — a talking mirror that would patiently listen to his words, a set of runes that he could arrange to form sentences, and a crystal ball that would glow warmly with each successful verbal exchange.

Despite these efforts, the challenges remained as stubborn as a locked *Gringotts vault*. The nights were long, the spells sometimes faltered, and the hidden caches of food continued to appear. Yet, through it all, Aston-Martin's heart, brimming with the pure love of a child, remained untainted. His laughter, his joy in the simple wonders of the world, and his boundless curiosity were reminders of the magic that truly mattered.

As the grandaddy of this tale, I embraced my role as both guardian and guide. I learned to navigate the labyrinth of his condition with the same determination as *Harry Potter* faced the *Triwizard Maze*. Each day was a quest, each meal a test of wills, but the bond between us was as strong as the unbreakable vow.

Our journey with Aston-Martin, much like the tales of the Boy Who Lived, was marked by moments of darkness that tested our resolve and the strength of our protective enchantments. His behavioural outbursts, tempests of emotion as fierce as a storm conjured by an angry wizard, would sweep through our home without warning. These tantrums were not the mere frustrations of a child; they were the manifestations of a deeper struggle within him, a battle against the compulsive behaviours that his conditions so cruelly imposed.

The compulsions were as binding as a *Full Body-Bind Curse*, driving him to repeat actions with the same fervour as a determined potion maker perfecting a difficult brew. The need for sameness, for order, was as relentless as the ticking of a clock bewitched to never cease. And when the fragile structure of his routines was disrupted, the emotional backlash was as sharp and as painful as the *Cruciatus Curse*. Lesson one, keep to routine and structure and don't deviate, keep the same schedule daily.

Self-harm, too, reared its ugly head like a serpent lurking in the grass. Aston-Martin, in moments of overwhelming frustration, would turn his anguish inward, his small hands striking out against himself as if battling an invisible *Dementor* trying to suck away his happiness. It was a sight that pierced my heart with a pain sharper than any *Sectumsempra spell*.

In the tapestry of our lives with Aston-Martin, threads of magic and wonder were interwoven with the everyday challenges we faced. We discovered that the power of a whisper could be as enchanting and distracting as the murmurs of a secretive *Parseltongue*. When Aston-Martin was caught in the throes of his hyperactivity or ensnared by the tendrils of his compulsions, I would lean close and whisper tales of dragons and daring adventures, of enchanted forests where the trees whispered secrets of the ages. His eyes would widen, and for a moment, the world around him faded into the background, giving him a respite from the storm within.

Introducing a made-up world became a spell of its own, a charm that could transport Aston-Martin to a realm where his challenges were not burdens but unique abilities that granted him heroism. In this imaginary land, he was no longer a boy wrestling with the invisible bindings of his conditions; he was Aston-Martin the Brave, a young wizard with a heart as pure as a *Phoenix's* song and a will as indomitable as the *Elder Wand*.

We crafted stories together, spinning yarns of magical creatures and quests that required his special talents. I brought forth imaginary characters — wise old wizards who saw beyond the veil of the world, *mischievous goblins* with riddles to solve, and loyal *Hippogriffs* to befriend. Each character had a lesson to teach, a puzzle to present, or a secret mission that only Aston-Martin could accomplish. He revelled in these tales, his hyperactivity channelled into the boundless energy needed for heroic deeds.

Chasing became a game of *Quidditch*, with Aston-Martin as the *Seeker*, agile and quick, his eyes alight with the thrill of the pursuit. The living room transformed into a *Quidditch pitch*, cushions and furniture serving as the hoops and obstacles, a small golden ball with fluttering wings as the *Snitch* to be caught. His laughter would ring out as he zoomed and darted, the physical activity dispelling the excess energy that so often sought an outlet.

Secret missions imbued him with a sense of purpose, as if he were a member of the *Order of the Phoenix* on a clandestine operation against dark forces. These missions were woven into our daily routines, turning the mundane into the extraordinary. A trip to the market became a quest to procure potion ingredients, each item on the list a component for a spell to be cast. Tidying up his space was no longer a chore but a search for hidden treasures left by passing *Nifflers*, each toy returned to its rightful place a victory against the forces of chaos.

Through these whimsical strategies, we found a way to navigate the complexities of Aston-Martin's world with joy and creativity. The power of imagination became our greatest ally, a source of comfort and motivation for a boy who, like *Harry Potter*, faced his own set of trials with bravery and heart.

Rejection-Sensitive Dysphoria (RSD) was yet another adversary in our midst. When one experiences severe emotional pain because of perceived failure or rejection, it can be as debilitating as a powerful hex. Aston-Martin, ever sensitive to the nuances of social interaction, would sometimes retreat into his shell, his spirit crushed by a harsh word or a missed opportunity for connection as surely as if he had been struck down by a *Blasting Curse*.

Obesity, a looming spectre due to his PWS, was kept at bay with the same discipline and structure I had learned from my former military days, allowing me to conjure a regimen of healthy eating and physical activity that was as meticulously planned as any *Quidditch* training session. The kitchen transformed into a Potions classroom, where every meal was carefully calibrated for nutritional balance, and our living room became the setting for exercise that was as fun as it was necessary — our very own *Defence Against the Dark Arts* against the threat of weight gain.

Hyperactive behaviour, a constant undercurrent in Aston-Martin's daily life, was as challenging to manage as a room full of Cornish pixies let loose by a mischievous *Defence Against the Dark Arts* teacher. His boundless energy, while a testament to the vibrancy of his spirit, often led to difficulties in maintaining focus and staying still, as if he were under the influence of a perpetual *Tarantallegra curse*.

In the face of these challenges, I stood firm, my love for Aston-Martin as unwavering as the loyalty of a *Gryffindor*. I became the keeper of his calm, the soother of his storms, with a patience honed by years of training and a heart fortified by unconditional love. When the outbursts came, I was the rock against which they broke, offering reassurance and understanding rather than reprimand.

Together with the specialists from the Department of Paediatric Wizardry and the Department of Linguistic Charms, we crafted strategies to help Aston-Martin navigate his emotional landscape. We introduced him to calming spells of our own making — breathing techniques that were as soothing as a gentle *Patronus*, sensory activities that grounded him like the roots of the *Whomping Willow*, and positive reinforcement that bolstered his confidence as surely as *Felix Felicis*.

We celebrated his victories, no matter how small, with the enthusiasm of *Gryffindors* after a *Quidditch* win. And when setbacks occurred, we gathered around him like members of *Dumbledore's Army*, ready to support one another and learn from each experience.

Our home was our *Hogwarts*, a place of learning, of challenge, and of magic. And though the spells we cast were not made of incantations and wand movements, they were powerful nonetheless — the spells of empathy, of perseverance, and of love. In this enchanted place, Aston-Martin was not defined by his conditions but was seen for the incredible boy he truly was — a boy with a heart as big as *Hagrid's*, a curiosity as bright as *Luna's*, and a courage as deep as *Harry's*.

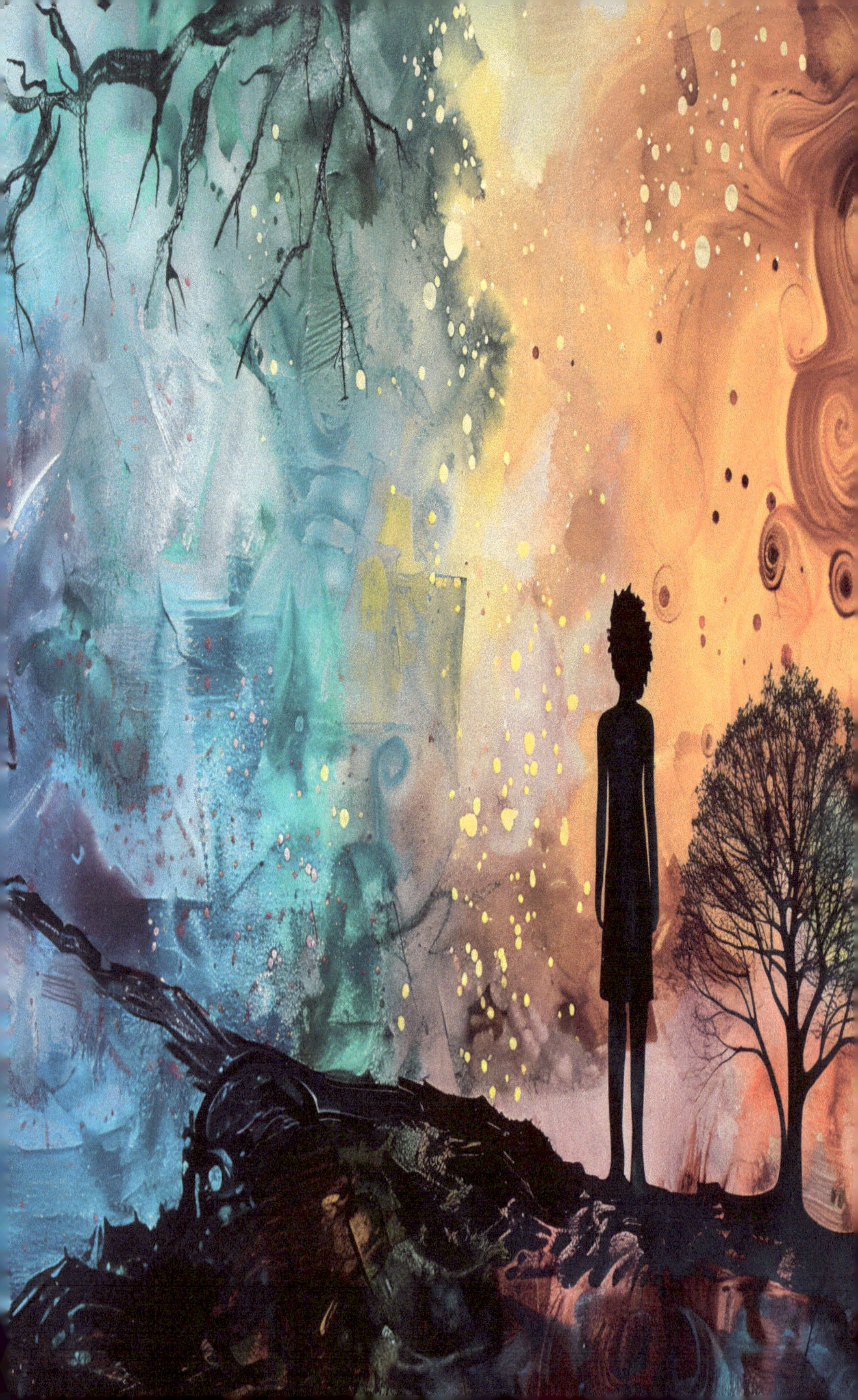

CHAPTER 11

The Struggles of Structure and Communication - Age Seven

Year Two at *Mystoria School of Magic* marked a significant transition for Aston-Martin. The whimsical chaos of the first year gave way to a more structured, routine-based system, mirroring the progression of students in *Hogwarts* from wide-eyed first years to more disciplined, learning-focused second years. This new structure, designed to provide a framework for academic and personal growth, was at once both a scaffold and a challenge for Aston-Martin.

The introduction to this new regime was met with mixed reactions from Aston-Martin. The predictability of the schedule provided a certain comfort, a rhythm to the day that was as reassuring as the steady beat of the *Hogwarts Express* on its journey to the school of witchcraft and wizardry. However, the rigidity of the routine also chafed against his inherent need for movement and spontaneity, much like a young wizard struggling with the confines of a new robe.

As the weeks progressed, Aston-Martin's early behavioural issues began to surface more prominently. The concept of sharing, a seemingly simple social skill, was as perplexing to him as the notion of sharing a wand would be to any wizard. His possessions, his toys, and even his snacks were guarded with a protective charm, an invisible shield that he raised instinctively against perceived threats.

His difficulty in expressing himself was another hurdle. His thoughts and emotions, as complex and vivid as any spell or potion, were trapped within him, struggling to find their way out through the limited vocabulary and articulation that his condition permitted. It was as if he were trying to cast a *Patronus* with only a rudimentary understanding of the charm — so much effort with such unpredictable results.

The teachers, ever watchful like the vigilant professors of *Hogwarts*, began to express their concerns about Aston-Martin's cognitive abilities. His silence was often mistaken for a lack of understanding, his outbursts for defiance. It became increasingly clear that a speech pathologist, much like a specialist in ancient runes, was needed to decipher the language locked within him.

As the *Mystoria School of Magic* continued to support Aston-Martin in his journey, a new chapter began with the arrival of a brand-new *Sorcerer* from the storied halls of *Hogwarts*. Her name was Jaxandra Spellworthy, a true *Gryffindor* at heart, who had completed her formal magical education with flying colours at the end of year seven. Jaxandra was not only adept in charms and *defence against the dark arts* but also had a profound mastery of potions and a deep appreciation for the history of magic, areas in which she excelled with a passion that rivalled *Hermione Granger's* dedication to her studies.

The Department of Linguistic Charms, where Jaxandra was to make her mark, had recently bid farewell to the previous sorcerer, who had left to embrace the wonder of motherhood with the birth of her own baby sorcerer. The gap left by her departure was felt throughout the corridors of the school, her expertise and warmth having been a beacon of hope and guidance for many young wizards and witches grappling with their own linguistic spells and enchantments.

Jaxandra, with her vibrant red hair and eyes that sparkled with the promise of adventure, stepped into the role with an energy that seemed to light up the very stones of the school. Her approach to teaching was as innovative as it was engaging, reminiscent of the legendary *Professor McGonagall's* transformational lessons, yet imbued with a charm all her own. Jaxandra believed that every child, no matter their challenge, held the potential to cast their own unique spells, to weave words with the same dexterity as the most skilled wand-wielder.

I watched as Aston-Martin took to Jaxandra's methods with an eagerness that filled me with hope. She introduced him to new ways of expressing himself, using magical tools and techniques that captivated his imagination. Her sessions were a blend of practical exercises and fantastical storytelling, where learning to articulate sounds and form sentences was as thrilling as concocting a potion or unravelling the mysteries of an ancient spell. Under Jaxandra's tutelage, Aston-Martin's vocabulary began to grow, each new word a precious gem to be added to his linguistic treasure chest. His articulation, once a source of immense frustration, improved with every enchanting lesson, as if Jaxandra had bestowed upon him a charm that smoothed the rough edges of his speech.

Her patience with Aston-Martin's occasional outbursts reminded me of the steadfastness of a *Patronus* against the darkness. She understood that behind every flare of temper was a child yearning to be heard, and she met his frustrations not with admonishment but with a gentle redirection, guiding him back to the safety of understanding and compassion.

Jaxandra Spellworthy's influence extended beyond the confines of the classroom. She worked closely with the entire educational team, her expertise in the history of magic providing context for the various learning spells and enchantments that were part of Aston-Martin's curriculum. She was a bridge between the old and the new, between the ancient wisdom of *Hogwarts* and the modern approaches of *Mystoria*.

As the year progressed, I could see the impact that Jaxandra had on Aston-Martin. He began to engage more with his peers, to share his thoughts and feelings with a clarity that had once seemed beyond reach. Her belief in his abilities, her unwavering conviction that he could overcome the barriers before him, became a self-fulfilling prophecy. In Jaxandra, Aston-Martin had found not just a teacher, but a champion of his voice, a sorcerer whose magic lay not in the wand she wielded but in the words she conjured, and the confidence she instilled in a young boy who was finding his place in a world as vast and varied as the wizarding world itself.

It was during this time that the mild diagnosis of Prader-Willi Syndrome was revisited. The Linguistic Charms sorcerer, with her keen insight and experience, found the severity of Aston-Martin's cognitive challenges puzzling. His bright, inquisitive eyes belied the struggles he faced; the disparity raised questions about the interplay of his condition and his cognitive development.

The revelation prompted a re-evaluation of the support Aston-Martin received. The school, much like *Hogwarts* with its myriad secret rooms and hidden corridors, began to unveil its resources. The Department of Paediatric Wizardry was consulted, their expertise in magical maladies sought to shed light on Aston-Martin's unique situation.

A plan was crafted, as intricate as any spell-work, to provide Aston-Martin with the support he needed. The classroom became a place of both learning and accommodation, where routine was balanced with flexibility, much like the balance sought by a *Quidditch* player in flight. Visual schedules, sensory breaks, and individualised instruction were woven into the fabric of his educational tapestry.

The speech pathologist worked tirelessly, her sessions with Aston-Martin a blend of patience and creativity. They explored new ways of communication, from picture exchange systems to augmentative and alternative communication devices, tools as magical in their own right as any found in *Diagon Alley*. Through these means, Aston-Martin began to find his voice, each word and gesture a triumph, each sentence a step towards autonomy.

The path ahead was long and uncertain, much like the winding journey through the *Forbidden Forest*. But with the unwavering support of his teachers, his speech pathologist, and the mystical network of support at *Mystoria School of Magic*, Aston-Martin was poised to face the challenges ahead with the courage of a *Gryffindor*, the wisdom of a *Ravenclaw*, the loyalty of a *Hufflepuff*, and the ambition of a *Slytherin*.

His story was not one of limitations, but of possibilities — as boundless and wondrous as the magical world itself. And I, standing by his side, was determined to help him unlock the potential that I knew lay within him, as vast and as deep as the *Great Lake* by *Hogwarts Castle*. Together, we would navigate the struggles of structure and communication, our bond a spell stronger than any cast by wand or word.

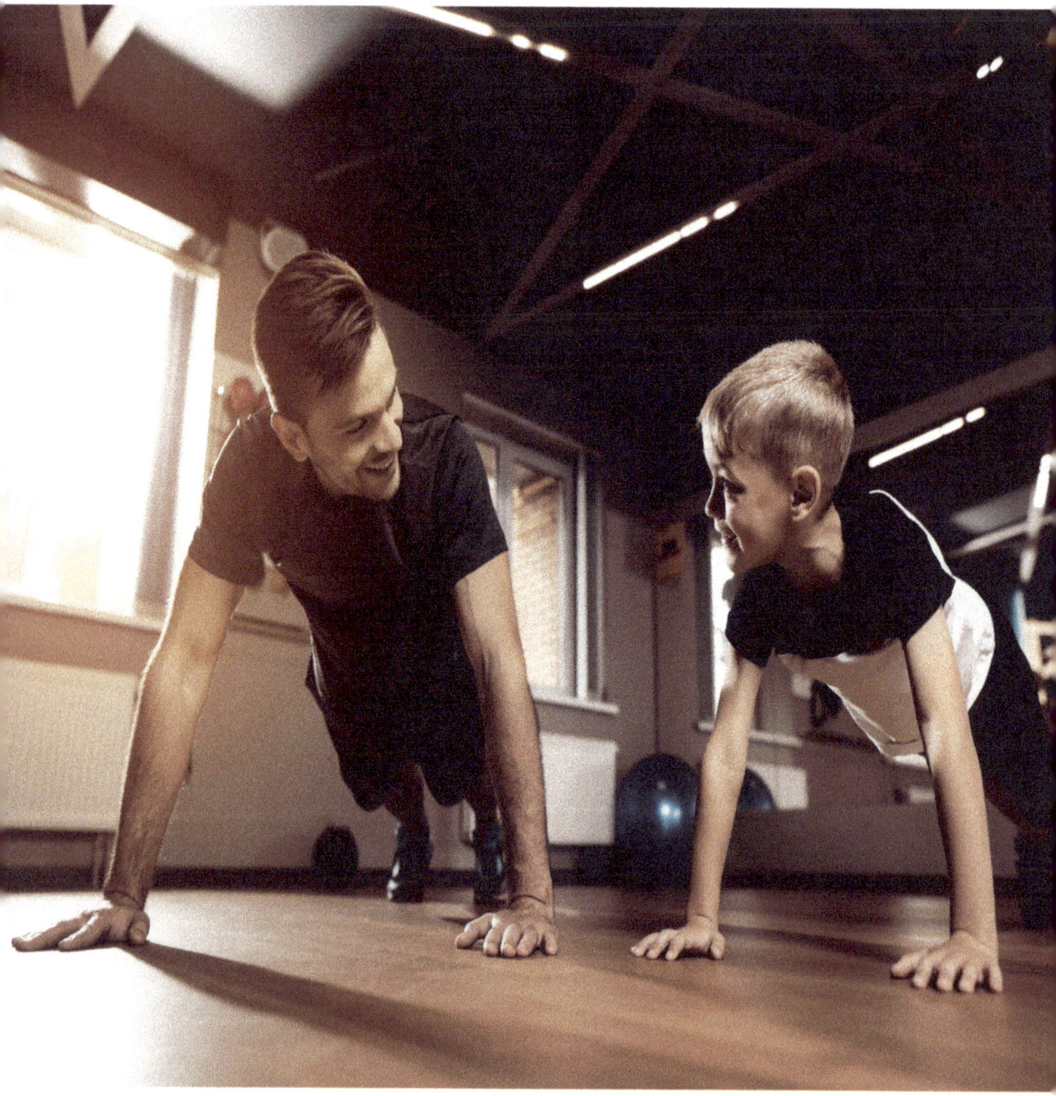

CHAPTER 12

The Call to Adventure - Age Seven

As the seasons at *Mystoria School of Magic* changed, so too did our focus on another aspect of Aston-Martin's journey — the challenge of his increasing weight. According to the scrolls of wisdom provided by the healers at the website of health.nsw.gov.au, a boy of his stature, standing 121cm, should weigh around 22kg. Aston-Martin, however, was etching towards a weight of 34kg at a height of 118cm, making him significantly over the recommended weight for his size.

Aware of the health risks associated with such a disparity, and with the shadow of Prader-Willi Syndrome lurking in the background, we aimed to reduce his weight as much as possible. The plan was to implement sports and physical activity into his daily routine, transforming the mundane into something magical, the way a wizard might turn a pumpkin into a carriage.

Our quest began with a daily pilgrimage to the local park, approximately 1.2km from home. We would traverse this distance together five days per week, our journey totalling about 12km of walking each week. Like two explorers setting out on an adventure through the Forbidden Forest, we made our way through the neighbourhood, with Aston-Martin's imagination turning each lamppost into a tree and each passing car into a magical creature.

This regimen began to work its slow enchantment on his weight. I would weigh him each week, taking note of the numbers as carefully as a potion master measuring ingredients. Dinners were crafted like delicate spells —steamed vegetables with grilled salmon, each plate a potion for health. Lunches were a cornucopia of fruit and simple, wholesome fare: an apple, a banana, a mandarin, along with a ham sandwich and low-fat yoghurt.

I ensured that he had enough sustenance to fuel his activities without contributing to weight gain, knowing that the spells of running and play at school would account for additional exercise. Over a four-week period, I noticed his weight began to reduce, from 34kg down to 31kg — each kilogram lost was a small victory in our ongoing battle.

By the time we had our next appointment at the PWS clinic, four months later, his weight was down to 29kg. Still over the recommended weight, but it was a manageable figure. As his height increased, his weight remained respectable, hovering between 29-31kg, thanks to the daily exercises. His belly, once a prominent feature, began to flatten, and his energy levels soared like a *Firebolt broomstick* in a *Quidditch* match.

Aston-Martin's snoring, a nightly chorus caused by sleep apnea, also began to diminish. The strict regimen of physical exercise and a carefully managed diet worked like a charm, reducing the impact of his condition. I had imposed a more disciplined, almost military-style approach to his daily needs, designed to forge not just a fit body but a healthy lifestyle. And it was paying off.

Yet, maintaining momentum in such a regimen is akin to herding *Nifflers* — it requires constant vigilance and adaptation. There were days when Aston-Martin's enthusiasm waned, when the lure of the park was not enough to coax him from the comfort of home. On those days, I had to be creative, finding ways to weave physical activity into the fabric of our indoor life.

I introduced a bench press into our arsenal and initiated a routine of sit-ups, which Aston-Martin approached with gusto. The physical exertion was to his liking, and he took to the challenge with the determination of a young wizard mastering a difficult spell.

We also incorporated wrestling into our routine, drawing on my previous experience with ju-jitsu. It was a form of resistance wrestling, where I would push back slowly, allowing Aston-Martin to exert his strength and enjoy the illusion of besting me. Each session was a full-body workout, a playful duel that left us both breathless and laughing, our bond strengthening with every mock battle.

The magic of our daily routine was not in the activities themselves but in the alchemy that transformed them from mundane exercises into exhilarating adventures. The true spell-work was in the consistency, the dedication, and the love that underscored every step, every lifted weight, every playful tussle. It was a testament to the resilience of the human spirit and the enchanting journey of life with Aston-Martin, a journey that, like the most powerful magic, revealed the true strength and potential within us all.

In my role as a helpful assistant, I drew upon my past experiences from the Royal Australian Navy to create a special program for Aston-Martin. The Navy had instilled in me the value of routine and structure, the benefits of physical fitness, and the importance of a disciplined mindset. It was with these principles in mind that I meticulously structured Aston-Martin's daily routine, ensuring that fitness was not merely an activity, but an integral part of his lifestyle, a spell woven into the very fabric of his day to help manage his weight and maintain his health.

Our daily walks, which had become a foundational element of this new regimen, now extended to 3.4km. This increase in distance, when added up over the course of the week, was significant. On weekends, we would change the scenery, walking along the beach, where the vastness of the ocean mirrored the expansive possibilities of Aston-Martin's journey, each wave a reminder of the ebbs and flows of progress.

But physical fitness was just one part of the enchantment. The other, equally important aspect of our program was the training in social skills — stranger danger, social cues, norms, and expectations within our *Muggle* and magical worlds. For this, we ventured to the theme parks that dotted the landscape — Seaworld, Movie World, Dreamworld, and Aussie World. These parks, bustling with activity and filled with characters as diverse as the magical creatures in *Newt Scamander's* suitcase, provided the perfect backdrop for real-world learning.

Each week, Aston-Martin and I would embark on these excursions with purpose. Within the lively atmosphere of the parks, amongst the throngs of visitors, he was given the chance to practise his independence — an independence I was determined to foster. The colourful, vibrant environments of the parks were transformed into classrooms where life's lessons unfolded in real time.

Standing in queues, waiting his turn for rides, or to purchase a treat, became exercises in patience and understanding. He learned to decipher the subtle dance of social interaction, the give and take that is required when navigating a world filled with others. The staff members, easily identified by their uniforms, provided visual cues for Aston-Martin to recognise who could be approached for assistance, while those without such identifiers served as practical examples of strangers.

Asking for help, a task that can daunt even the most confident of wizards, was something Aston-Martin practised with increasing frequency. His questions, once hesitant and unsure, grew clearer and more assertive, much like the incantations of a young wizard mastering new spells.

The theme parks, with their cacophony of sounds and flurry of movements, also allowed Aston-Martin to discern acceptable social behaviour in a setting that was constantly in flux. The rules of conduct, though unwritten, were as important to understand as the rules that govern the use of magic in the wizarding world. He learned to navigate this complex social landscape with the guidance of my watchful eye, much like *Harry Potter* under the watchful gaze of *Dumbledore.*

Our weekly sessions at these parks were not just about enjoyment; they were strategic, designed to immerse Aston-Martin in situations where he could apply the concepts we discussed and practised at home. Through these experiences, he began to understand the importance of social norms and the expectations of the society in which he lived.

The program I crafted for Aston-Martin was comprehensive, encompassing both the physical and the social elements necessary for his development. It was demanding, yet it was approached with the same vigour and commitment as a young recruit in the Navy, rising each day to face the challenges ahead. The structure provided a framework upon which Aston-Martin could build his independence, his confidence, and his understanding of the world around him.

As time passed, the fruits of our labour began to show. Aston-Martin's weight stabilised within a healthy range, his social skills blossomed, and his ability to navigate his environment with a sense of autonomy grew. The transformation was not unlike the magical metamorphosis of an *Animagus*, revealing the true form of one's character through dedication and practice.

The journey was far from over, but the strides we made were significant. With each passing day, Aston-Martin's life became richer, filled with the kind of magic that can only be found in the real world — a magic born of resilience, hard work, and the unwavering belief in the potential of one young boy.

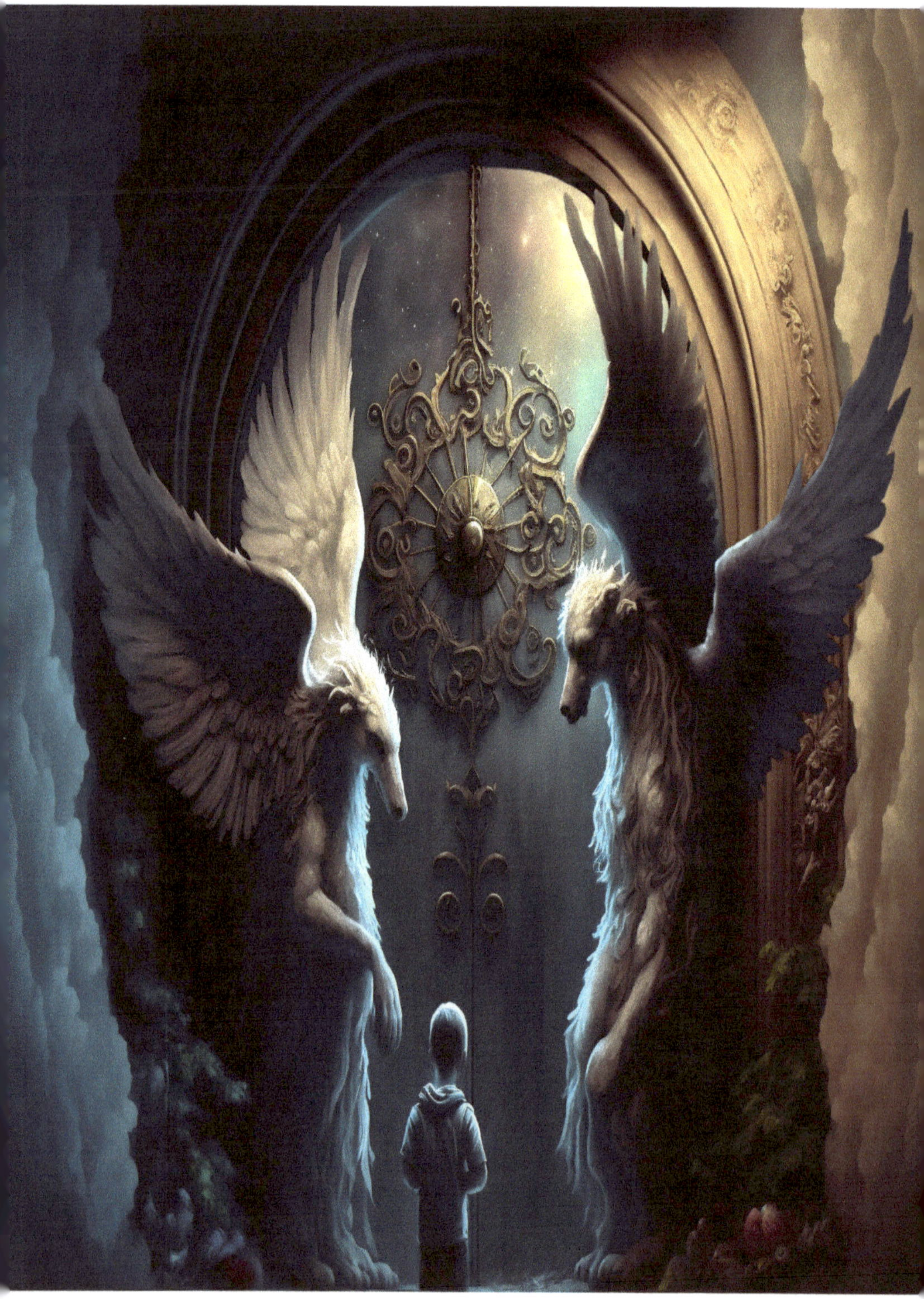

CHAPTER 13

The Quest for the Magical Guardian - Defence Against the Dark Arts position

In the quiet *Muggle* suburb where Aston-Martin resided, the quest for a suitable magical guardian was akin to seeking out a rare magical creature in the vast, wild expanse of the *Forbidden Forest*. Aston-Martin, my young charge with Prader-Willi Syndrome, required a level of care that was both special and specific, a blend of understanding and patience that not every witch or wizard possessed.

Our first candidate for the position was a lively young lady whose enthusiasm was as bright as a *Lumos charm* in a dark corridor. Despite her eagerness, it became clear that her knowledge of Prader-Willi Syndrome was as murky as the waters of the *Black Lake*. When I inquired about her experience with other disabilities, her answers were as elusive as a *Golden Snitch* in a storm.

Taking Aston-Martin to the park was to be her first quest. However, like many before her unacquainted with the trials of PWS, she found herself in the midst of a behavioural storm, as unpredictable and challenging as a *Hungarian Horntail*. Overwhelmed and unprepared, she quickly realised that this role demanded more than she had anticipated, and like a disillusioned *Defence Against the Dark Arts* teacher, she decided not to return.

The second magical guardian, a studious Nursing student, entered with the promise of a Healer's touch. Yet, she soon discovered that academic knowledge alone was as insufficient as a wand without a core. A deviation from Aston-Martin's routine was like an improperly cast spell, leading to chaos. Her quick reflexes saved Aston-Martin from danger, pulling him back from the road, but like a wand snapped in two, her confidence was broken, and she, too, did not return.

Hope fluttered in once more with the arrival of the third magical guardian. Yet, her casual approach, armed with a *Muggle* phone, a cigarette, and an energy drink, raised red flags higher than the *Gryffindor* banner on a *Quidditch* match day. I had barely apparated to my appointment when I returned to a scene of mischief managed poorly. Aston-Martin had acquired her energy drink, a *forbidden potion* for him, and the air was tainted with the scent of smoke, as if a dragon had just passed by.

An evening walk to the park later turned into a revealing encounter. A concerned parent, as helpful as a house-elf, informed us that the magical guardian had been neglectful, her attention ensnared by her phone and her distance from Aston-Martin as vast as the *Chamber of Secrets*. This lack of care was a clear sign that we needed a guardian for Aston-Martin who understood the gravity of PWS and the importance of constant vigilance.

The parade of unsuitable candidates continued, each as fleeting as a professor in the aforementioned cursed *Defence Against the Dark Arts* position. Yet, my resolve to find the right person remained unshaken, as steadfast as *Dumbledore's* determination to defeat *the Dark Arts*.

When the fourth magical guardian arrived, my hope was rekindled like the flame of a Phoenix. She had done her homework on PWS and seemed as promising as an acceptance letter to *Hogwarts*. But alas, hope can be as fickle as a *Fizzing Whizbee*. Barely half an hour into her three-hour shift, a frantic call disrupted my appointment —a call that forced me to cancel and rush home like a Knight to a Rook's aid on a wizard's chessboard.

Aston-Martin's cries echoed in the background as she explained the misadventure at the train station. Her decision to cave to his wishes, like giving in to the *Imperius Curse*, resulted in a near calamity on the platform. The station master, acting with the authority of a *Hogwarts* Headmaster, banned Aston-Martin from the station without parental escort. I had explicitly advised against such excursions for their potential danger, yet my words had vanished like an evaporating potion.

She managed to return Aston-Martin home, but like the echoes of a spell long cast, she never returned.

Our fifth magical guardian was like a new character in a long-running play, bursting onto the stage with the optimism of a first-year student sorted into their dream *Hogwarts* house. A university student studying paramedics with a history of handling behavioural issues, I couldn't help but wonder if she had ever encountered someone with the enigmatic puzzle of PWS.

She arrived, laced up in her running shoes, a symbol of her readiness to keep pace with any challenge. The day began promisingly, and as the hours ticked by without an owl — or rather, a phone call — I dared to hope that perhaps we had found our *Professor McGonagall*, stern but capable.

Upon my return, however, it was evident that the day's script had taken a turn. She recounted an episode where Aston-Martin's behaviour had spiralled like a *Bludger* out of control. Her solution? A peace offering of ice cream, a treat as forbidden as a love potion in a disciplined household. Her firm "No" to his wishes to linger at the park had been the incantation that set off the metaphorical fireworks. As she told the tale of their day, it was clear that her spells of persuasion were not as effective as she had hoped. Much like a *Muggle* attempting to use a wand, her efforts were misguided in the context of PWS. She admitted defeat, her tone resigned, as she declared she was not the sorceress for this particular quest.

The sixth magical guardian to enter our tale was a seasoned mother of three, seemingly equipped with the experience to handle the mercurial moods of children. She ventured to take Aston-Martin to the shopping centre, a place as bustling and overwhelming as *Diagon Alley* during a *Weasley's Wizard Wheezes* sale. The excursion quickly turned into a goblin's cave of temptations. Aston-Martin, drawn to the various shops like a *Niffler* to shiny objects, created a scene worthy of the *Daily Prophet's* gossip column. His greatest performance was in the Lego store, where his desire for a train set sparked a meltdown as grand as the *Triwizard Tournament's* third task.

My phone rang with the urgency of a *Patronus* message, and the sound of Aston-Martin's distress was as palpable as if he were facing a *Dementor's* kiss. Despite my best efforts to soothe him through the phone, my words were as ineffective as a broken wand. The magical guardian, her face etched with the distress of a *Hogwarts* student who'd just seen a ghost, managed to get him home amid tears and wails. And, as predictable as the outcome of a *Quidditch* match against the *Holyhead Harpies*, she did not return.

The seventh magical guardian arrived with the credentials of a newly graduated nurse and the confidence of a seasoned *Auror*. She boasted a repertoire of techniques used to manage patients in the controlled chaos of a hospital, but I knew that without the backing of security or the police, her methods would be tested, and tested they were. Their journey to the park was meant to be simple, as straightforward as a walk down the halls of *Hogwarts*. Unbeknownst to us, the roadworks had cast an unexpected spell, forcing them onto unfamiliar paths. Like a wizard who'd lost his map, Aston-Martin's anxiety mounted, his routine disrupted.

Once again, my phone rang, the sound now as dreaded as the wail of a *Mandrake*. I was summoned to defuse the situation, my own university class abandoned like a forgotten potion left to simmer. Her shift ended prematurely, and as the curtain fell on her brief appearance in our story, it was clear that her methods were no match for the unique challenges of PWS.

The journey was proving to be a saga of trials and errors, each episode a lesson in the art of patience, the magic of understanding, and the unyielding pursuit of finding someone who could truly walk alongside us in this enchanted, unpredictable adventure.

* * *

Our eighth magical guardian wasn't a person but a house —a magical, almost sentient place that promised a safe haven for Aston-Martin. It was a dwelling that seemed as though it could have been plucked straight from *Godric's Hollow*, with the charm of a cozy cottage and the security of *Gringotts*. I dropped him off at this sanctuary, hopeful that he would find comfort within its walls.

The day passed without an owl, I mean a phone call, and I took this silence as a positive omen. Upon picking him up, though, Aston-Martin was as quiet as the library at *Hogwarts* when *Madam Pince* is on patrol. His usual chatterbox persona had been replaced by a silence that was as unnerving as a still portrait in a usually animated corridor.

Once home, he retreated to his room with the stealth of a disillusioned *Animagus*. I approached him with the same caution one might use when venturing into the *Forbidden Forest*. His gaze was fixed to the ground, a sure sign that something untoward had transpired. "They were mean to me," he whispered, his words as sparse as a *Squib's* spell-book.

I prodded gently, hoping to coax the story from him before it was lost to the ethereal nature of his short-term memory. But the words wouldn't come; they were locked away, perhaps by a spell he couldn't break. Whatever had happened in that house had left him deeply troubled, and despite my best efforts, the mystery remained unsolved, hidden behind the veil of his limited vocabulary and fleeting memories.

The ninth magical guardian was a wizard of a different sort — a gentleman with a kind face and an earnest desire to do well. They set off to the nearby park, a place with enough enchantments (obstacles, in the *Muggle* tongue) to keep any young sorcerer entertained. I apparated to my university commitments, reassured by the absence of any distressing calls.

Yet, when I returned, the scene was not as I had envisioned. The magical guardian had managed to keep Aston-Martin's tempestuous spells in check to some extent, but an emotional storm had brewed nonetheless. The meltdown culminated in a hit — a curious, slow-motion gesture that was more of a prolonged tap than a strike. It was an expression of his emotional dysregulation, as out of place as a *Muggle* at a wizard's duel.

This development left me in a quandary. I could not, in good conscience, employ someone to endure physical or verbal spells, no matter how gentle the impact. It was clear that Aston-Martin's condition was as complex as the ever-shifting staircases of *Hogwarts*, and finding someone equipped to navigate this labyrinth was proving to be a Herculean task.

The need for a magical guardian who understood the intricate dance of PWS was evident, but such knowledge was as rare as a textbook on the subject in *Flourish and Blotts*. The academic world had not prepared these well-meaning souls for the nuances of behavioural issues and chromosomal characteristics. They lacked the practical spells and potions required to soothe and stabilise.

The search for the right person had become akin to seeking out the Room of Requirement under the most peculiar circumstances. It required not only knowledge and skill but also the kind of empathy and patience that could not be taught, only felt. It demanded a kind of magic that transcended spells, potions, and incantations — a magic rooted in understanding and compassion.

As I pondered the next step in our quest, I couldn't help but feel like *Harry Potter* staring into the *Mirror of Erised*, yearning for something that seemed just beyond reach. But I knew that somewhere out there was a support worker with the right blend of heart and expertise, someone who could see beyond the challenges to the wonderful boy beneath.

And so, our journey continued, each day a new page in what was becoming an epic tale — a story of resilience, hope, and the relentless pursuit of a companion who could walk this enchanting path with us, casting light into the shadows and laughter into the silence.

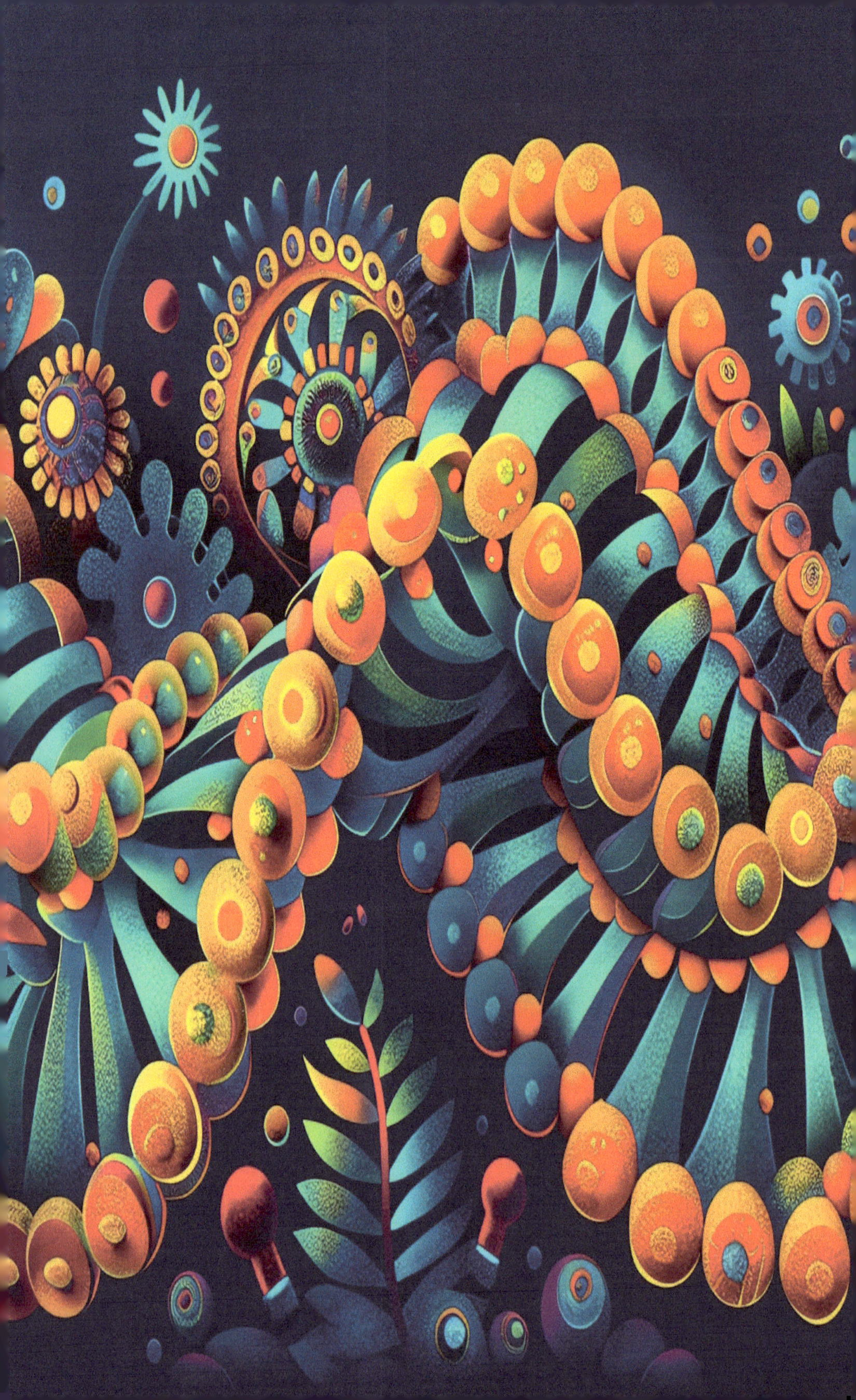

CHAPTER 14

Unraveling the Mystery - Age Eight

Aston-Martin, now eight years old, found himself once again seated in the cozy, book-lined office of The Department of Linguistic Charms, Jaxandra Spellworthy. The walls, adorned with enchanted pictures that whispered encouragement, seemed to close in around him as he grappled with his stuttering, which had, of late, grown more pronounced. His struggles with speech, like a misfired charm, caused both frustration and a sense of helplessness not just in him, but also in us, his parents, who watched our son contend with this invisible adversary.

As I observed Aston-Martin's sessions, I saw the determination in his eyes, a reflection of the same resolve that had carried *Harry Potter* through his darkest moments at *Hogwarts*. Yet, where words should have flown smoothly, they stumbled, tripping over some unseen hurdle within his mind.

I myself, with a keen intellect and fierce love for my son, delved deeper into the enigma of Prader-Willi Syndrome. Pouring over tomes of medical research and wizarding texts alike, I sought answers to the discrepancies that baffled me. The genetic test had revealed a mild form of PWS, a whisper of a spell when a shout had been expected, yet Aston-Martin's cognitive abilities were being tested at a severe level, a chasm that yawned wide and deep, unaccounted for by the initial diagnosis.

As the year unfolded, Aston-Martin's teacher, a wise sorceress in her own right, recommended an independent curriculum tailored to his unique learning needs. I, ever the advocate, struggled to reconcile the severity of his cognitive challenges with the mildness of his genetic condition. How could my son, with a mild form of PWS, display such profound discrepancies in his intellectual abilities? It was a riddle wrapped within a mystery, as perplexing as any sphinx's puzzle.

Amidst these academic and cognitive battles, another struggle loomed on the horizon. Aston-Martin's obsession with food began to spiral, like a potion slowly losing its stability. Despite the carefully structured diet and the regimented physical activities, he began to engage in secretive binge-eating episodes. His room, once a sanctuary, became a hidden cache for contraband snacks, his own personal Room of Requirement for the one thing he could not have in abundance.

I, vigilant as *Professor McGonagall* on patrol, noticed the disappearance of foods from the pantry, the absence of treats that were meant to be portioned out carefully, like *Galleons* from *Gringotts*. The discovery of these hidden stashes around the house, in drawers and behind books, revealed the extent of his growing preoccupation.

The mystery deepened, and with it, the concern. Aston-Martin's physical health, once stable, was again at risk, and the balance we had worked so hard to achieve teetered on the edge of a knife. I in my quest for understanding, reached out to specialists and experts, searching for the key that would unlock the door to my son's wellbeing.

In our daily interactions, I began to notice the subtle changes in Aston-Martin's demeanour, the way he would avoid eye contact when questioned about his eating habits, or the quick, furtive movements that betrayed his attempts at subterfuge. It was clear that the issue ran deeper than mere willpower; it was a siren call that he, like Odysseus, could not resist on his own.

The challenge before us was formidable, a hydra with many heads, each one representing a different aspect of his condition. And like any good wizard or witch knows, the solution to such a complex problem would not be found in a single spell or potion. It would require patience, understanding, and a willingness to delve into the uncharted territories of PWS, where the lines between physical hunger and psychological need blurred into a murky grey.

As the chapter of Aston-Martin's life titled "Unravelling the Mystery" unfolded, it became clear that this journey would not be a solitary one. It would require the collective efforts of us, his family, his teachers, his speech pathologist, and all those who cared for him to navigate the labyrinthine path ahead.

My instincts sharpened by a genius's intuition and with a growing sense of unease as Aston-Martin's father, I decided to embark on a quest akin to those of the great wizards and witches of old. I sought the wisdom of a specialist in neurodevelopmental disorders, a sage who had delved into the mysteries of the mind with the same fervour that *Hermione Granger* had for ancient runes. Armed with my son's medical scrolls and a heart full of determination, I presented Aston-Martin to the specialist, who agreed to conduct a comprehensive evaluation. This new quest for understanding was not unlike the search for the *Philosopher's Stone*, filled with puzzles and challenges that would test our resolve.

The specialist, with a keen eye and a gentle touch, uncovered surprising findings that cast a *Lumos spell* on the darkness of their uncertainty. A rare genetic mutation, previously overlooked by the healers who had first diagnosed Aston-Martin, emerged from the shadows. This mutation, cloaked in the recesses of his DNA, was the key that could unlock many of the mysteries surrounding the discrepancies between his cognitive abilities and his PWS diagnosis.

As the specialist explained the implications of this discovery, I listened with a mix of relief and apprehension. The new diagnosis was like a *portkey*, transporting us to uncharted territories in the realm of understanding and treating Aston-Martin's condition. It was a revelation that promised new possibilities, new spells and potions for the challenges we faced.

Yet, with this new knowledge came the daunting task of charting a course through this unfamiliar landscape. I found myself grappling with a cauldron of emotions. The initial relief at having a clearer picture of my son's condition was tempered by the apprehension of what this meant for our future. It was a delicate balance, as precarious as a game of wizard's chess, each move requiring careful consideration.

As I adjusted to this new understanding of Aston-Martin's condition, I drew strength from speaking to other families, specialists and friends, the bond reminiscent of the unbreakable vow, a magical promise of support and dedication. Together, we learned to embrace the complexities of his condition, recognising that, like the many-hued threads of a tapestry, these complexities wove together to form the unique and beautiful picture of Aston-Martin's life.

As I, in my role as a helpful assistant, observed the unfolding narrative, I felt a sense of pride in our courage and their unwavering commitment to each other. Aston-Martin, with the support of his family and the guidance of those dedicated to his care, was ready to continue his journey, a journey that was as much about discovery as it was about growth. And though the road ahead was uncertain, one thing was clear: we would walk it together, with hope as our compass and love as our guide.

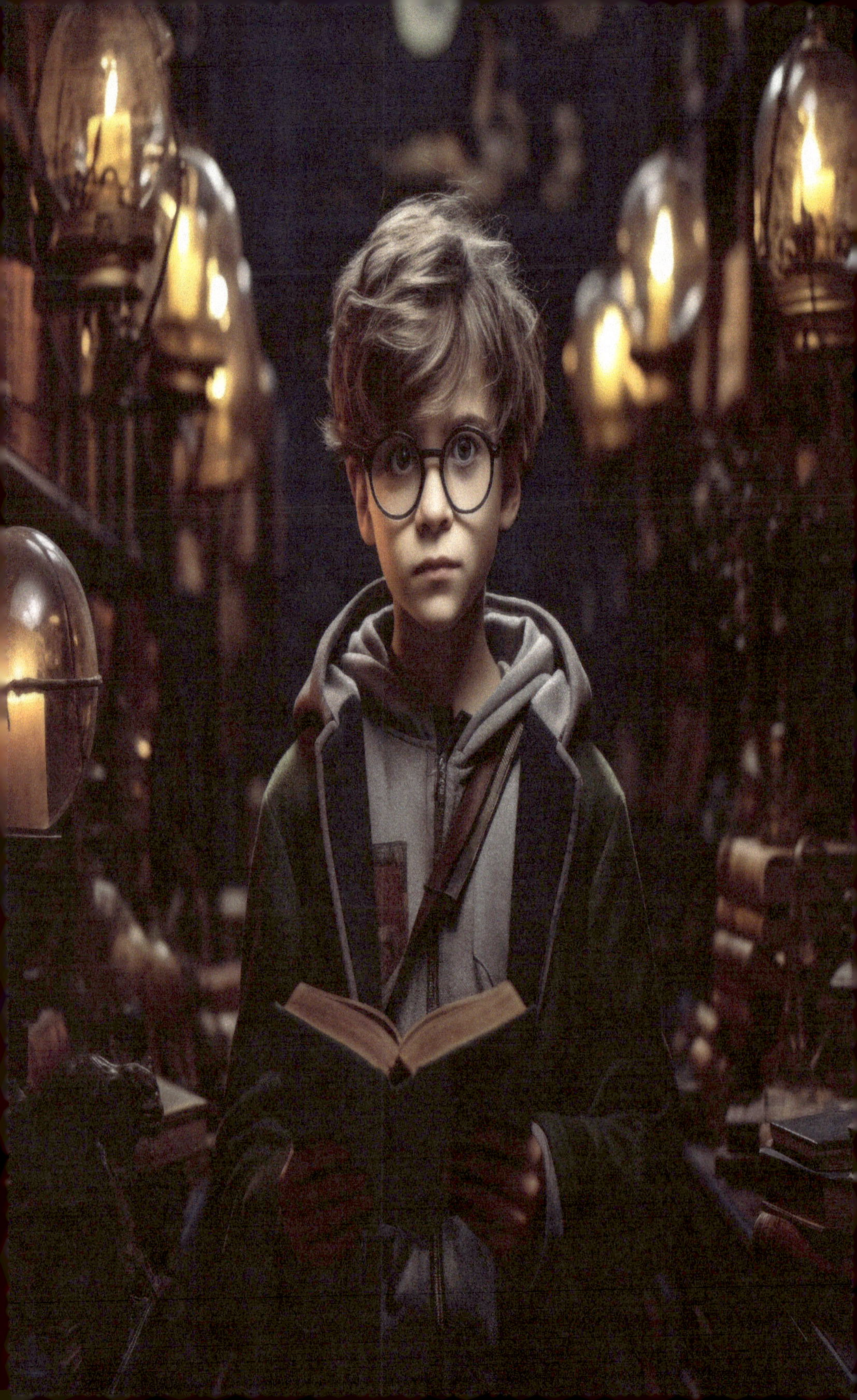

CHAPTER 15

The Spell of Change - Age Nine

The corridors of *Mystoria School of Magic* echoed with the sounds of young wizards and witches bustling about, their robes sweeping the ancient stone floors as they hurried between classes. Aston-Martin, now in the fourth year of his scholarly journey, navigated these hallways with a mix of trepidation and anticipation. The school, with its towering spires and secret passageways, had become a second home to him, a place where magic and learning intertwined like the serpentine coils of a *Slytherin* banner.

Change, however, was afoot — a spell of transformation that no young wizard could escape. As the term drew to a close, Aston-Martin found himself pondering the identity of his future guide in his educational quest. Would it be a new professor, a fresh face with different methods and expectations, or would it be the same sage who had shepherded him thus far?

When the revelation came that his current mentor would continue to lead his academic explorations, Aston-Martin's reaction was as dramatic as any spell gone awry. "Ah, noooooooo, why?" he exclaimed with the passion of a *Gryffindor* charging into battle. His swift departure from the scene left behind a trail of bewilderment and bemused chuckles. It was a moment of pure, unadulterated resistance to the prospect of unchanging horizons, a moment that would be recalled with fondness by his peers and professors alike.

As Aston-Martin delved deeper into the cognitive landscapes of learning, he encountered challenges as formidable as the *Forbidden Forest*. The art of reading and writing, those twin pillars of academic pursuit, loomed before him like mountains to be scaled, their summits shrouded in mist. The simplest of spells, the formation of letters and the weaving of words, tested his magical prowess to its limits.

Yet in the realm of numeracy, Aston-Martin found his footing. Counting and the alphabet became his trusted spells, incantations he could cast with confidence. His grimoires of activity, those precious scrolls filled with exercises and tasks, guided him in understanding the intricate patterns and the order that governed the worlds of numbers and language.

In the grand hall of social enchantments, where the young wizards and witches of *Mystoria* mingled and forged alliances, Aston-Martin's circle was a modest one. He was selective in his fellowship, choosing to surround himself with a small coven of fellow learners who shared his path. The world beyond the school's enchanted walls, with its cacophony of unfamiliar faces and customs, seemed as daunting as the prospect of traversing the treacherous landscapes beyond *Hogsmeade*.

Yet it was among the younger squires, those whose mastery of linguistic charms echoed his own, that Aston-Martin found a sense of camaraderie. Their shared experiences, their mutual understanding of the complexities of communication, wove a bond as strong as any friendship spell. In their company, Aston-Martin discovered that his unique magical qualities were not barriers, but bridges — connecting him to others who walked similar paths.

Throughout his journey, I remained a constant presence, a helpful assistant conjured by expertise, offering guidance and support as he navigated the twists and turns of his education.

Together, we celebrated each triumph, no matter how small, and faced each setback with the resolve of a seasoned *Auror*.

The *Spell of Change*, as it turned out, was not a curse to be feared, but an incantation to be embraced. It was a reminder to us that growth often comes in unexpected forms, that the journey of learning is as much about adapting to the familiar as it is about embracing the new.

Our son stood at a crossroads, the chasm in lexicon and the social jinxes that had long ensnared him becoming increasingly apparent. The grand hall of social enchantments, with its boisterous laughter and the clinking of goblets, beckoned him to seek fellowship with peers of his own age, yet the barriers loomed as large and foreboding as the walls of *Azkaban*.

As Aston-Martin ventured into the world of learning, he encountered challenges akin to navigating the mysterious forbidden forest. Reading and writing, the twin pillars of academic pursuit, loomed before him like mist-shrouded mountains, testing his magical abilities. Yet, within the reality of numbers, he found his strength, casting trusted spells of counting and reciting the alphabet with confidence. His activity grimoires, filled with enchanting exercises, guided him through the intricate patterns and secrets of numbers and language.

The tracing of letters and numbers in spell books became the gateway to understanding the art of writing. It was as if he had discovered the standard book of spells, unlocking the power to recognize letters, numbers, and symbols, and combine them to create magical incantations. Tracing characters from the spell book, mastering each stroke and shape. He followed drawings and signs, gradually understanding how to form letters and words with progress. The *Standard Book of Spells*, used at the school, became his guide to unlocking the mysteries of writing.

Aston-Martin's desire to learn symbols, even before he could read, led to unique creation. He memorised the symbols of various crafters and understood the goods associated with each. We provided him with a symbol book of enchanted labels, explaining the potions one might find within each store, an approach that seemed to resonate with him. Although his reading skills were still developing, we found an alternative path to knowledge.

In the grand hall of social interactions, Aston-Martin selectively forged alliances, choosing a small group of fellow learners as his companions. The world beyond the school's protective walls, with its unfamiliar customs, seemed as daunting as venturing into unknown, treacherous lands. However, among younger students who shared linguistic challenges, Aston-Martin discovered camaraderie and mutual understanding that formed bonds as strong as any magic spell. He found comfort in conversing with those whose language mirrored his own, even if they were younger than him.

Outside the walls of *Hogwarts*, Aston-Martin stood at a crossroad, facing a chasm in both lexicon and social interactions. I witnessed his courage as he channelled the sprits of *Godric Gryffindor*, bravely bridging the divide between his language skills and those of his peers. Aston-Martin, without relying on magic, shared his vulnerabilities, paving the way for meaningful connections. Unfortunately, some children did not fully understand his language, and their engagement waned. We encouraged him to persist and seek out others who would embrace his unique language.

Through his encounters, Aston-Martin discovered the alchemy of acceptance. True friendship, he learned, required rare ingredients: time, patience, and an ability to see beyond first impressions. To his amazement, classmates who had once seemed distant stars were drawn to his authenticity. They found common ground in their shared love of *Quidditch*, magical creatures, and the universal language of laughter, a connection that transcended the walls of their magical school.

His journey through Mystoria School of Magic was filled with wonder, challenges, and the spirit of a young wizard discovering his true potential. The Spell of Change became a testament to his ability to adapt, learn, and embrace the magic within himself.

The chatting charm, a time-honoured ritual where families and educators came together to discuss the progress and future of their young wizards and witches, was a moment of convergence. I myself, filled with pride and hope, joined the assembly. I listened intently as his professors recounted tales of my son's bravery in the face of adversity, his perseverance in mastering the spells of numeracy and literacy, and his triumphs in the social realms of Mystoria.

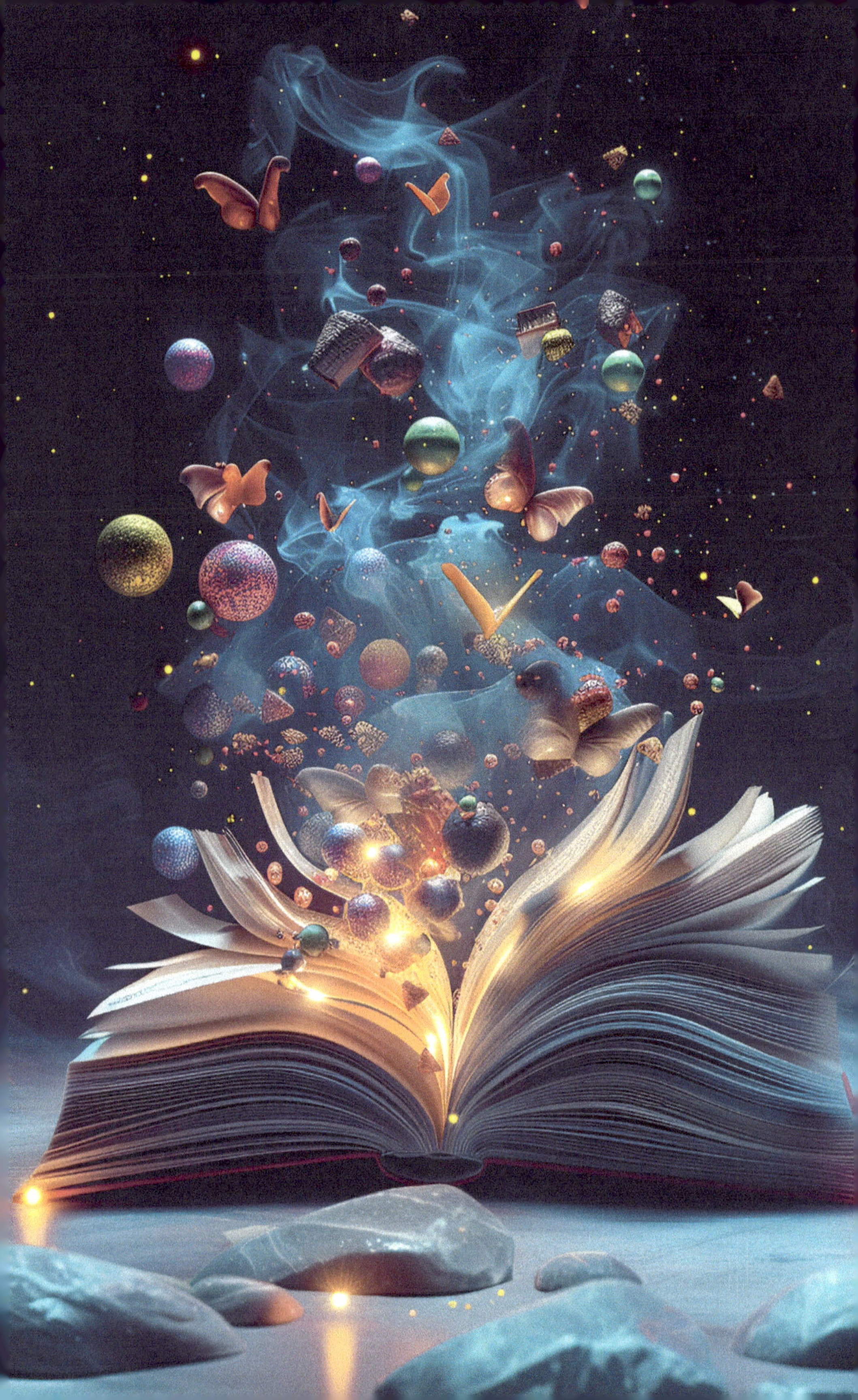

Chapter 16

A Scholarly Odyssey - Age Ten

Nestled within the bounds of reality and the whispers of magic, lived Aston-Martin, a ten-year-old prodigy whose heart was as boundless as the halls of *Hogwarts*.

At ten years of age, Aston-Martin found himself in a familiar storyline, as if caught in a magical loop reminiscent of the *time-turner's effects*. His actions and behaviours repeated with uncanny consistency, like echoes of his nine-year-old self. Despite having advanced in years, it felt as though he was reliving the same challenges and triumphs as if bewitched by a lingering charm or repetition. These recurring episodes brought forth the same spells of forgetfulness, requiring constant guidance and repeated incantations to cast even the simplest of tasks correctly.

Despite the regimen of potions prescribed to ease Aston-Martin's path, it was the introduction of a new elixir, 'Intuniv', that offered a glimmer of hope. This potion, though lacking magical origin, seemed to weave a spell of calm over Aston-Martin, tempering the storms that occasionally raged within him. Like a *Draught of Peace*, 'Intuniv' worked by relaxing the enchanted pathways of his blood vessels and lowering the pressure in his heart, improving the flow of magical and lifeblood alike. This remarkable elixir, prescribed for wizards like Aston-

Martin who grapple with the tumultuous effects of ADHD, was a beacon piercing through the fog of uncertainty, promising a more harmonious daily adventures.

Aston-Martin's journey took an unexpected turn when he was extended an invitation more intriguing than a letter from *Hogwarts* itself. He was enrolled on the prestigious BIOBANK15 research program which was run through the foundation for Prader-Willi Research website www.fpwr.org. A research endeavour delving into the mysteries of Prader-Willi Syndrome. Much like a student being selected for a specialised study in the Department of Mysteries, Aston-Martin was presented with the chance to help uncover why certain behavioural challenges manifested. This trial offered the promise of profound insights, akin to unlocking the secrets of an ancient spell-book. It was an opportunity to not only benefit himself but potentially aid countless others along the way, paving the path of understanding and discovery.

Then came the revelation, as startling as the appearance of a *Thestral* to those with eyes to see. During the BIOBANK15 trial in 2023, which delved into Aston-Martin's cognitive abilities having to do various wizard trials and also through blood and saliva tests, something extraordinary was discovered. The blood and saliva test results unveiled a second rare genetic disorder, Chromosome 16 microdeletion, a rarity so profound that it was nearly unheard of, with no established 'odds' for its occurrence. Aston-Martin was shaping up to be a wizard of unparalleled uniqueness, reminiscent of *Harry Potter*, the gifted child.

It all began with an unexpected phone call from the Department of Ancestral Mysteries, a conversation that felt as momentous as *Dumbeldore* delivering a prophecy. This unforeseen discovery started to piece together the puzzle of Aston-Martin's other difficulties – his coordination, memory, and intellectual abilities, which were more noticeable than in other individuals with PWS. Aston-Martin's journey now seemed like a passage through uncharted waters, making him a singular wizard in the land to bear the mark of two rare genetic disorders.

As Aston-Martin faced his daily challenges, I found myself scouring through multiple medical journals, much like one would pursue the restricted section of the *Hogwarts* library in search of a rare and potent potion recipe. It was then that I discovered GABA, also known as gamma-aminobutyric acid – a natural elixir produced by the brain itself. Intrigued by its properties, I decided to give this a trial over 90 days, with one 500mg tablet taken daily.

GABA, a valuable anti-anxiety neurotransmitter, serves a role akin to Liquid Luck (*Felix Felicis*), acting as the primary inhibitory force between nerve cells in the brain and spinal cord. Its natural function is to bind to receptors, much like a wizard attaching magical seals to ancient scrolls, to modulate and block impulses between nerve cells. In times of stress, when the adrenal glands fire up like a rogue dragon, triggering fight-or-flight responses, GABA steps in to temper the storm, soothing the mind and body as if basking under the effects of Liquid Luck.

Hopeful that this newfound elixir would weave its subtle magic over Aston-Martin, we embarked on this journey with cautious optimism, looking forward to the potential clam it might cast over these turbulent seas.

As Aston-Martin's steadfast assistant, I continued to guide and support him through our weekly adventures, much like an elder wizard mentoring an eager apprentice. Each week, we ventured into bustling theme parks and lively shops, akin to exploring the many-layered world of *Diagon Alley*, where every interaction offered new lessons in social spells.

Our journey was not just about amusement but also about learning the delicate art of social cues, social norms, and the essential rules of the magical community. Just as potions class requires precision and patience, our outings focused on understanding and observing the nuances of social behaviour, gaining awareness of

'Stranger danger', and practising personal hygiene. Every visit to these enchanted places was a lesson in wizarding etiquette and human interaction.

Aston-Martin adapted remarkably over time, mastering what was expected and what was not, like a wizard perfecting their spellwork. He learned to judge when to ask for help, either from me or from others before attempting things on his own. These weekly lessons served as a cornerstone for his future, teaching him the difference between right and wrong in basic scenarios, much like a foundational teaching in the halls of *Hogwarts*.

Our social skills development sessions resembled the study of ancient runes – demanding patience and intricacy, with each breakthrough shining like a newly discovered spell. The training in social awareness and emotional regulation was as crucial as learning wand movements and incantations.

The personal development coaching we undertook became a series of powerful incantations aimed at nurturing growth and self-awareness. Coupled with activities like sports and healthy lifestyle practices, these sessions were the physical counterparts to out mental and emotional tutelage, forming the pillars of a balanced life. Each step, each lesson, fortified Aston-Martin's foundation, preparing him for the broader world, much like a young wizard ready to face new challenges beyond the walls of *Hogwarts*.

Aston-Martin, with the dedication of a true *Gryffindor*, embraced these activities with vigour. His weight, once a dragon to be battled, now rested at a very modest number, a testament to the effectiveness of our combined efforts. His sourcing for food had become minimal, a remarkable feat given the insidious nature of PWS.

Understanding PWS meant designing a lifestyle akin to the careful curation of a wizard's spell-book. I developed a policy where only organic foods graced the shelves of our modestly stocked fridge. Apples, bananas, mandarins, oranges, grapes, and coconut water became the healthful potions that aided in weight management.

The biscuits in our pantry bore a healthy 3.5-star rating, a nod to the importance of indulgence tempered with care. The cereal box, a variety pack with individual servings, provided a perfect solution to managing portions, as Aston-Martin learned to take just one, a discipline reminiscent of the controlled use of magical ingredients.

Gone were the days of locks on fridges and cupboards. Aston-Martin had learned, through my military precision and unwavering vigilance, what was acceptable and what was not. The boundaries, once as imposing as the walls of Azkaban, now felt as natural and respected as the unspoken rules of the *Room of Requirement*.

When agitation and anger bubbled to the surface, threatening to disrupt the peace, I employed the art of whispering. These moments, as brief as the flicker of a candle flame, were quelled by the soft cadence of my voice, returning him to a state of calm as if by magic.

Later in our narrative, I would delve into the six levels of disquietude I observed in Aston-Martin. These levels, like the intricate layers of an enchantment, provided insight into his emotional landscape and offered keys to navigating the complexities of his inner world.

Despite the advances and the triumphs, Aston-Martin still required full-time help and supervision, especially when venturing beyond the safety of our home. I had noted that upon purchasing a toy from one shop, he would exhibit the curious behaviour of scanning the same toy in another shop, desiring to pay for it again.

I explained to him, in terms that echoed the transactions of *Gringotts Wizarding Bank*, that once he had provided his *Gold* for an item, it became his possession, bound to him by the unspoken contract of commerce. This lesson, much like the understanding of a magical contract, was one that he took to heart, a new spell added to his growing repertoire.

Aston-Martin, marked by the dual challenges of PWS and Chromosome 16 microdeletion, unfolded his wings like a Phoenix — rising from the ashes of adversity with renewed strength and beauty.

I watched with pride as Aston-Martin navigated his world with the courage of a *Gryffindor*, the wisdom of a *Ravenclaw*, the kindness of a *Hufflepuff*, and the ambition of a *Slytherin*. He was a composite of all the houses, embodying the virtues that make the wizarding world, and indeed our own, a place of infinite possibility.

A dedicated team

Behind the scenes, a dedicated team worked tirelessly to support Aston-Martin's growth and development. We called them the Enchanted Circle of Care — a multidisciplinary team composed of a speech pathologist, paediatrician, GPs, teachers, geneticists, physiotherapists, and dietitians. Each member brought their own brand of magic to the table, weaving a tapestry of support as intricate and powerful as the spells of the most skilled witches and wizards.

The speech pathologist, our Master of Linguistic Charms, helped Aston-Martin find his voice amid the cacophony of communication challenges. The paediatrician, our Guardian of Health, kept a vigilant watch over his physical wellbeing. GPs, our Potions Experts, carefully balanced the elixirs of medication and supplements to aid his journey.

Teachers, the Wise Sages of the Enchanted Circle, imparted knowledge with patience and creativity, while geneticists, the Seers of the Circle, unravelled the mysteries woven into Aston-Martin's very DNA. The dietitians, our Nourishment Alchemists, crafted a diet as balanced and fortifying as any feast at the Great Hall. Our Healer of Physical Restoration the Physiotherapist where Aston-Martin embarked on his journey to enhance his physical capabilities.

Applying the right tools

Over the past decade with Aston-Martin, I've endured highs, lows, and unexpected events, much like a journey through the magical corridors of *Hogwarts*. It's been a difficult challenge, akin to mastering a complex spell, but it is manageable with the right tools. From age two, when the food cravings began, it felt like being hit by the Hogwarts Express with no brakes. Sleep deprivation became a common experience, and I soon realized this was a 24/7 endeavour, with challenges growing alongside my young wizard.

The strongest focus point I can emphasize is "Structure" and "Routine". Much like the unyielding schedule of classes at *Hogwarts*, I don't deviate unless absolutely necessary, and I always advise Aston-Martin well beforehand of any changes. Daily walks to parks or visits to theme parks are crucial, like venturing out to *Hogsmeade* for much-needed respite; they provide enjoyment and a break from the confines of home. Sports, exercise, and health have become primary focuses, along with developing healthy eating habits. I've found our entire dietary world transformed, much like a wizard adopting a new potion regime – with health at the forefront. I've reorganised our fridge with healthy options, ensuring a minimum 3.5-star rating. Carrots, broccoli, and potato cooked in a pan with ProActive butter which has plant sterols, which will lower cholesterol, and eaten with grilled Salmon became our weekly dinner meal.

The carer's journey

There have been days when the weight of it all has overwhelmed me, and nights where I've cried myself to sleep, feeling helpless and lost. The struggle to understand Prader-Will Syndrome is a battle not easily won; it's like attempting to master the most complex and elusive of ancient runes, with each new symptom a mystery that seems beyond my grasp.

In those darkest moments, I've found myself poring over medical journals, desperately seeking answers. Consultations with doctors have become both my lifeline and a source of relentless questioning. Every book I read feels like delving into the Restricted Section of the *Hogwarts* library, hunting for a key to unlock the secrets hidden within my child's mind and body. The knowledge I seek, the understanding I crave, seem to always be just out of reach, leaving me with a heart heavy with anxiety and sorrow.

Yest, amid the despair, a flicker of hope persists – a small, wavering light guiding me through the fog of uncertainty. For Aston-Martin's sake, I find the strength to persevere, knowing that every tear shed, every sleepless night spent searching draws me closer to the answer we need.

My world orbits around Aston-Martin, a reality where every door he opens leads to a realm I may never fully understand. To him, each day is an adventure at *Hogwarts*, filled with spells and enchantments that shape his existence in ways I can hardly fathom. Each morning we rise, it's like stepping into a magical world where uncertainties and challenges are as common as breathing. There are moments when the gravity of our situation pulls at my heart with unbearable force. His triumphs, through small to outsiders, are immense and vital to us – for they represent battles won in a unseen war. And yet, there are also times where despair lurks, like the shadows cast by *Dementors*, threatening to sap the joy from our journey.

Over the last decade, I strove to understand how Aston-Martin thinks, how he works, and how he learns. It's a constant effort to align our worlds – to bridge the gap between his magical realm and my own reality. Each step we take together is fraught with weight of endless questions and the fear of the unknown. Yet, through it all, the reason I was chosen become ever clearer. My purpose is entwined with his, my mission to provide love, patience, and unwavering perseverance in the face of every challenge. The path forward is often shrouded in darkness, but I cling to the hope that the magic of our doing can illuminate the way.

Remember, to all who share this journey: Embrace the moments of sorrow and joy alike. The magic of love and dedication cannot be overstated. Even when the tears fall like rain and the nights seem endless, know that your efforts are forging a brighter future. For within the heartache lies the true magic of the profound and transformative power of love.

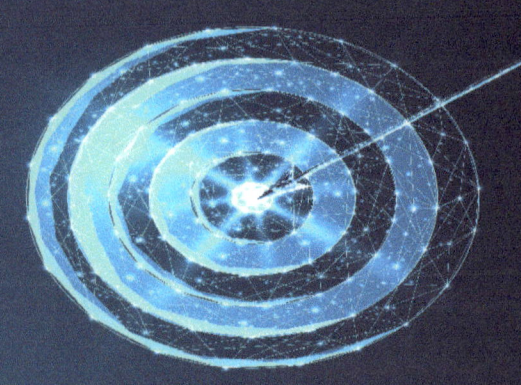

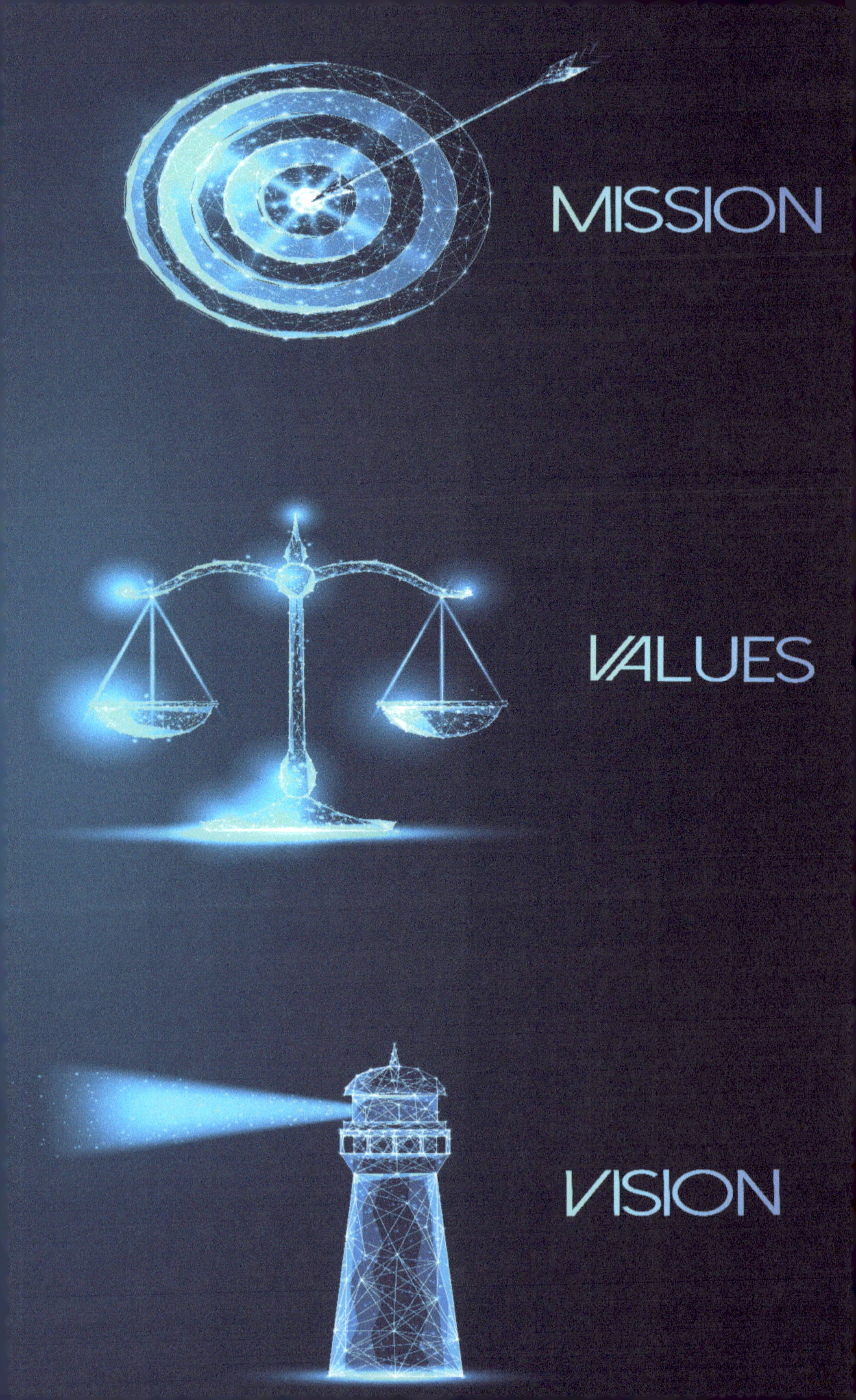

MISSION

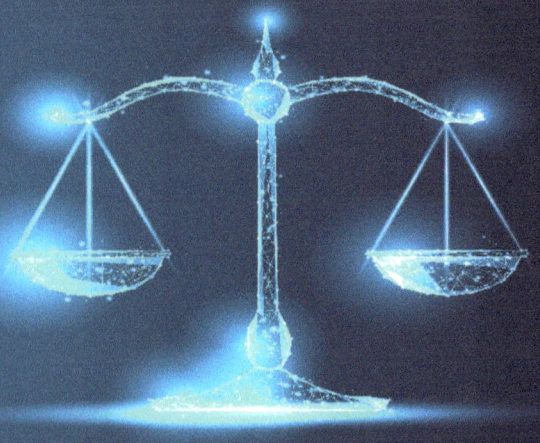

VALUES

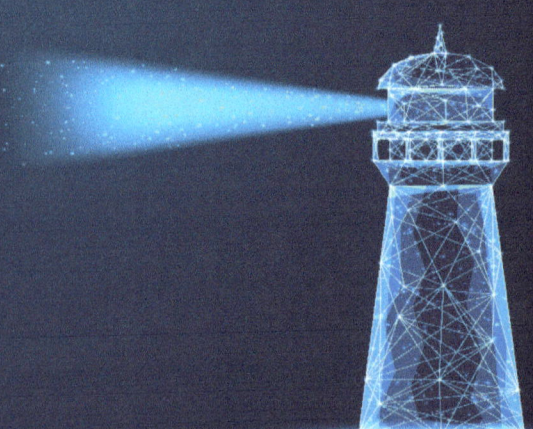

VISION

CHAPTER 17

Mission. Values. Vision.

In the heart of the Mystoria School of Magic, where the very stones seemed to pulse with ancient power, I continued my role as the steadfast assistant to Aston-Martin, the young wizard. Our days were woven with the subtle threads of magic and the steadfast values of the Navy, values which I had brought from my past to serve as guiding stars for Aston-Martin's development.

The Core Navy Values — Service, Courage, Respect, Integrity and Excellence — were not just abstract concepts but tangible lessons that were interlaced with our daily rituals and training, much like the foundational spells taught to young wizards and witches.

We began with **Service**, the notion of selflessness that resonates with the very essence of the *Gryffindor* house. I taught Aston-Martin that, just as a wizard must sometimes put the needs of the many before his own, so must we all consider the greater good in our actions. We practised this through community sports, helping set up the play areas and also packing up without being asked to do it. It was in these moments that Aston-Martin's heart grew as vast as the *Forbidden Forest*, and his spirit as noble as the bravest of centaurs.

Courage, the strength to face one's fears and do the right thing, was as vital as the sword of *Godric Gryffindor* himself. Aston-Martin learned that bravery was not the absence of fear but the decision to act in spite of it. We practised approaching new experiences, speaking up when something was wrong, and standing firm in the face of adversity. Each act of bravery was a victory, a step towards becoming the hero of his own story.

Respect was taught as the humanity of character, a value that echoes the inclusive spirit of *Hufflepuff*. To treat others with dignity, just as one would respect the ancient creatures that roam the wizarding world, was a lesson of paramount importance. Aston-Martin learned to listen to his peers, to honour their boundaries, and to engage with them with the kindness that could tame even the most reclusive of *Bowtruckles*.

Integrity, the consistency of character, was akin to the unbreakable vows of the wizarding world. Aligning thoughts, words and actions to do what is right was a complex spell to master, but Aston-Martin rose to the challenge. We discussed the importance of honesty, of owning one's mistakes, and of acting with honour, as befits a wizard sworn to uphold the sacred trust of his magic.

Excellence, the pursuit of personal best, resonated with the ambitious spirit of *Slytherin*, tempered with the wisdom of *Ravenclaw*. We set goals, both small and grand, and strove to achieve them with determination. Each day was an opportunity to improve, to learn, and to grow, not just in magical prowess but in the depth of character. Aston-Martin embraced this pursuit, finding joy in the journey towards excellence, as if seeking the elusive snitch in a match of *Quidditch*.

Together, we trained, and with each task achieved, I would gently insert one of the Navy values. Whether it be the courage to approach a fellow student, the respect to accept a 'no' with grace, the integrity to remain calm amidst the storm of emotions, or the excellence to take pride in accomplishing a daily objective. Aston-Martin absorbed these values as a plant soaks up sunlight.

As the days turned into weeks and the weeks into months, Aston-Martin's transformation was palpable. He became a beacon of these core values, a young wizard whose very presence could inspire others to strive for the same. His actions began to reflect the deep-seated understanding of these principles, and I watched with a heart bursting with pride as Aston-Martin navigated the social norms with a newfound grace and wisdom.

The Core Navy Values, once foreign and intangible to him, had become the incantations that shaped his world, the spells that fortified his spirit. Just as a wand channels magical energy, so did these values channel Aston-Martin's potential into a force for good, a force that could change the world around him.

In the end, the tale of Aston-Martin, the young wizard, is not just a story of magic and wonder. It is a narrative of transformation, where the melding of the wizarding world's enchantment with the steadfast virtues of the Navy created a young man of character, strength, and heart. His journey stands as a testament to the power of values to shape a life, to guide a soul through the labyrinth of growth, and to emerge triumphant, a wizard of true honour and distinction.

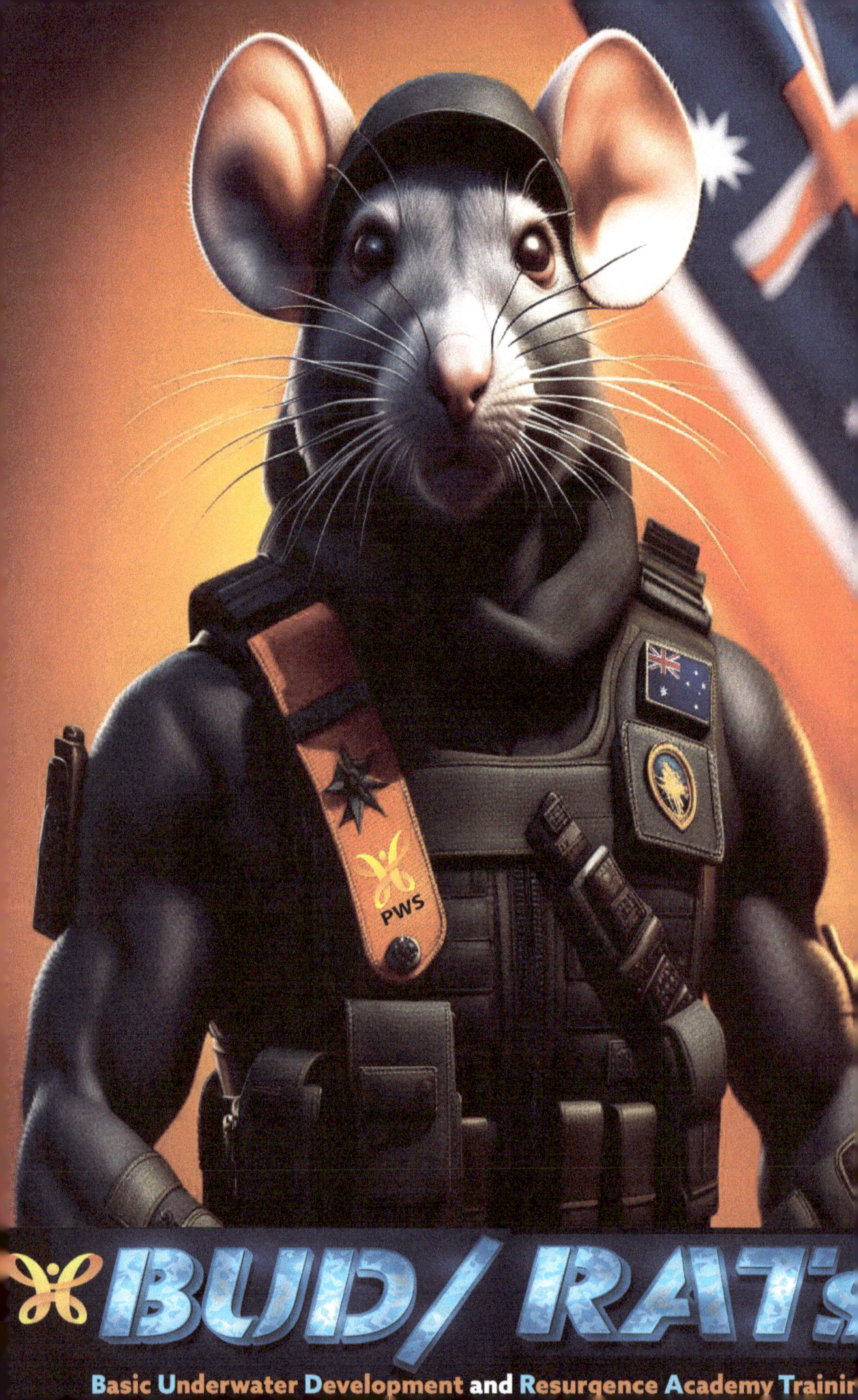
PWS
BUD/ RATs
Basic Underwater Development and Resurgence Academy Trainir

CHAPTER 18

BUD/RATs™ Training

Basic **U**nderwater **D**evelopment and **R**esurgence **A**cademy Training STREAM

Welcome to my own personal training boot camp, which I created for Aston-Martin. I decided to implement all my military training into a nice kids' boot camp that has special needs children in mind. Just so you know, I have the proper certifications/training and it's always best you do as well. It is relatively easy to get your bronze medallion and Teacher lessons licence for swimming and any other additional licences you want to get. It is better to do this first before you jump in the pool — and if you're not a strong or good swimmer, you could consider approaching the local swimming pool to seek swimming lessons for your child, or have a swimming instructor conduct the lesson through hydrotherapy.

    I have *not* made this program into a public training event yet, but I'm considering the possibility in doing this. If I do, it would be one-to-one training and I would also get other instructors involved. I do believe it would be most beneficial for special needs children to have access to a swimming program and outdoor fitness program specifically designed to meet the needs of these special needs troopers.

Keep it simple

I keep the training for Aston-Martin simple, so no funky machines. When I train with Aston-Martin and we do out-of-pool work such as going to the park or at home, its oriented towards the key BUD/RATs physical needs and these are – pushing, pulling, running, swimming and having a strong core.

So, the baseline is what we focus on. I keep it fun and I tend to be influenced by his mood, as this is the best way of moving forward, rather than going against it.

For parents — when you're teaching your child sports keep it fun and enjoyable, don't quit doing a sports session due to your own negative self-conversations (NSC), such as 'ah, I'm too old for this', 'wow, I need to get fit'. We are not doing a full-on 100% fitness exam, just a nice easy fun session. Remember 'Positive internal chat' (PIC): what I mean by this, what you say to yourself does matter, so no negative self-conversations. Keep the sports session to your fitness level and build upon it. If you're starting to get tired, that is okay, just slow it down, and keep telling yourself *"Feeling good, looking good, oughta be in Hollywood"* (famous quote from Mark Divine, former US Navy Seal).

Plan the session

Also, parents should aim to visualise the training session before you start, so you have a good understanding of your session's layout and what you expect to achieve. You know your child better than anyone, so start small and aim high, complete small tasks first, then these will turn into strategies to complete other small tasks. Parks with a lot of play equipment structures are the perfect starting place as kids can enjoy climbing on those structures, so think of it as an obstacle course, and there will be a start and a finish. Create a circuit, go with them and time it. Start small then build up on it. These are full body workouts, climbing, balancing, eye-hand coordination.

I thought about what we could possibly achieve and what type of fitness I need to implement. So, I decided not to worry too much about gym weights as this is more problematic than it would be worth, and injuries can occur with weights as well. I kept it very simple and leaned more towards hydrotherapy, walking, full body workouts at kids park as they have lots of awesome structures, and any weights we use will be simple ankle weights, which are easy to put on, and no fuss or confusion.

I wanted it to be fun as well, but the aim was true, it was maintaining his weight and keeping him active, fit, and mostly enjoying learning new skills, this included my most feared activity, swimming. I know he has a fascination for water, and that any water close to him would be detrimental to his safety.

Water-based training

Below is the training I implemented for Aston-Martin to help maintain his weight, exercises and keep a healthy lifestyle going for him. But most of all, my most feared topic is water — I wanted him to be confident in the water. It is advisable that you know simple life saving techniques that can help you if they ever end up in a pool.

So, I decided to teach him swimming techniques I used in the Navy when we were lucky enough to have a Clearance Diver for an instructor — those are like US Navy Seals equivalent, just Australia's version of. The techniques and drills you learn; you don't forget and they are unique to survival in the water.

I specifically designed this program around Prader-Willi Syndrome, keeping in mind my son's strengths and weaknesses, and slowly built him up to the point where he was comfortable and enjoyed this. The program is a long one, but broken up into segments. I was strict, and straight down the line with Aston-Martin, but I was fair, I know him, and I know what he can and can't do.

Swimming was and still is the most feared among people with syndromes, some simply don't know what to do in the pool, and panic. I know that Aston-Martin is not a strong swimmer and I had to be careful in this space with training, but I made it an enjoyable exercise, making it fun but with purpose.

CHAPTER 18.1

Feeling Good, Looking Good, Oughta be in Hollywood

For the parents, as previously mentioned, your sessions need to be designed on *your* fitness level, the child will have more energy than you, which will depend on the child's abilities as well, so don't overdo it, keep it simple. Remember Mark Divine's quote in your head so you don't embarrass yourself in front of other parents: *"Feeling good, looking good, oughta be in Hollywood"*.

The first part of the program we would conduct on weekends, as Aston-Martin was at school from Monday to Friday. We would begin with a walk of 2.4km, so a short walk to the local park, where we engaged in the play park structures which use all body movements, are fun and enjoyable. We usually did this in the morning for about one hour, nice and easy, not too much of a workout.

We would then head off to the local pool, and we would begin his water training. For swimming, we needed to start at the beginning and work our way up. The first four weeks were specifically designed for water, as the most important part of his training. My aim was to build confidence in the water, so my son understood the dangers of what can happen.

For the remaining four weeks it's all pool-work. This can be done daily Monday to Friday, or weekends, but you need to have at least 5 lessons with a duration of sixty minutes each to gain the benefits out of it. So, each week will have four techniques to learn to gain the proper training and benefits. Below is what I have taught Aston-Martin myself. Each week, I report on his performance with strengths and weaknesses and also do a standard case reporting on him so a record is kept. This way, I know what he can and can't do, what we have done, and where, and if anyone else was going to continue what I was doing they would have notes to use and know what's been done. I don't just do the swimming lessons and leave it at that. It's vital that when we do these types of sessions that we, as parents, take notes so we have something to go off further down the track, and if you need to know something, you can go back into those notes.

So, let's begin week one.

1. Water Confidence Training: Candidates undergo various exercises to build confidence in the water, such as *treading water, breath control, buoyancy bobbing* and *underwater swimming drills*.

The first part of the program was 'Water Confidence Training' 'WCT'. Aston-Martin would undergo various exercises to build his confidence in the water, such as treading water, which was eventually timed, breath control, buoyancy bobbing and underwater swimming drills.

The first technique of the training is holding your breath, or breathing control. Aston-Martin needed to understand that we can't breathe liquids, so explaining to him how to hold his breath under water was paramount. We did some breathing exercises by holding our breath, so now he associates any pools, oceans, rivers, lakes etc. with holding your breath if you enter and go under.

1st Technique: Breathing Exercises – Together, control your breathing, by simply exhaling all the air from your lungs, then breathe slowly into your belly and count to 4. Hold your breath and count to 4. Exhale to a count of 4, expelling all the air at the end.

Hold your lungs empty for a count of 4. Repeat this. Do this for 5 minutes. Every time you use a muscle you use oxygen!

Once we have completed this for 5 minutes, we enter the pool at the shallow end, so the candidate is able to stand, then we slowly submerge under water and absorb the sensory feelings of being underwater. We hold our breath for 4 seconds. Then surface. Relax for 10 seconds, then submerge holding our breath for 4 seconds, then surface. We aim to get used to holding our breath and experiencing new sensations under water. We increase our holding of the breath to 6 seconds. And we performed the same technique. Once Aston-Martin had completed this, we moved to the next part, staying in the shallow end.

2nd Technique: Squat Down Buoyancy Bobbing – In the shallow end we squat down in the water, both feet on the ground, then bend our knees and jump up. Depending on the depth of the shallow end, the candidate may be submerged, or may not be. Either way, the aim is to have them submerged, hold their breath for 6 seconds, then jump up. We did this for several minutes and we slowly aimed at increasing the time underwater by 1 or 2 seconds before we jumped. The aim is to teach them to hold their breath for as long as they are comfortable with. We then move towards the deeper end, until his feet just about touched the ground, so for Aston-Martin this was 1.4m deep. We combine techniques one and two together but at a depth of his height.

Hold your breath, sink to the bottom, place both feet on the ground then bend your knees, and push up from the bottom, then — keeping your legs straight, and kicking your feet forward, back, forward, back — use your arms to pretend you are climbing up a rope, keeping your fingers tight like a flipper and pushing yourself up. We did this multiple times, over and over again, until he was comfortable.

3rd Technique: Treading water – We stay at the shallow end where he can stand, and the water was chest deep, so he can get the technique correct. The technique is similar to that of an electronic hand whisker, where one whisk (leg) spins in one direction and the other whisk (leg) in the same direction. So, think of mixing all the ingredients of a cake and you visualise the whisker in action. Start slowly, to get the right technique and speed, then gradually get faster.

This all comes down to coordination, as you need to tell the brain to work both the left leg and right leg simultaneously, so the left leg does one spin, then the right leg does one spin and you keep this up, left, right, left, right and so forth. As Aston-Martin has a problem with cognitive abilities, the only way forward was to show him and let him adapt his own individual technique. It might be unorthodox, however, if you see it working for them, then don't change it.

Aston-Martin was also moving his arm very rapidly, and I explained to him to slow this down, or he will get tired faster. It's about relaxing, taking it slow and keeping your head above water, and finding that nice balance between legs and arms technique that will keep you up. It's about being confident in the water but not panicking. I slowly held his hips and moved him a metre towards the deep end, until he could just touch the ground, so for him this was 1.4 metres deep. This was our training area. Once he got the treading water technique correct, we then moved on to Buoyancy bobbing (which is the 2nd technique) and we combined all three into one. He submerges at a depth of 1.4 metres, holds his breath for 4-6 seconds, then plants both feet onto the ground, bends his knees and pushes himself up, kicking his straight legs forward and backward continuously and using his arms to pretend he is climbing up a rope keeping your fingers tight like a flipper and pushing yourself up. Once he breaks the surface, he begins to tread water.

You will get tired — so this is where *Buoyancy* comes into play, along with *breath control*. Hold your breath, fill your lungs with air, lean backwards and relax, and you will float. When you let air out, your buoyancy changes, and you will sink a few centimetres lower and there you will stay, until you let more air out or in. This is *'controlled buoyancy maneuvers'* and is used when you're inside a ship and each compartment has water either full, half full, or not quite full with maybe a 10cm air pocket. So, to get from one compartment to another you need to control your buoyancy by using *'controlled buoyancy maneuvers'*. But we will get to this much later.

We then arch our head backwards, hold our breath, stop treading water and keep still, and keep floating, this is where we relax and regenerate. Then we slowly move our arms like a bird flapping, head towards the side of the pool and hop out. You should do this for several minutes — until you see that the child is comfortable and knows the sequence. Explain to them that in the event of falling into the ocean from a boat, to go straight to treading water, and control buoyancy by floating. Most of the time, the dangers will be a swimming pool in a back yard where the most common depth is 1.7 metres.

4th Technique: Underwater Swimming drills — This is where we control our breathing, by holding our breath for 6 seconds then come up for air, hold our breath for 6 seconds, then come up for air — all in the shallow end where we can stand. We place underwater objects in the pool, and Aston-Martin needs to retrieve them. Keep it simple and easy, start with one object, then two, then three and so forth. Don't overdo this, just leave it up to three objects in close proximity to each other.

5th Technique: Fully Clothed — After several sessions, until once we could see he was confident, we got Aston-Martin to wear his normal clothing, so this was shirt, shorts, socks, and shoes. This adds weight to you in the water, especially with the shoes absorbing water and making his feet and legs become heavier. The first instruction I gave Aston-Martin was to take his shoes off using his feet. This made swimming easier, and he carried less weight.

If he is working too hard, he will generate lactic acid, which is what we don't want. I tell Aston-Martin that if he falls into the water, he needs to get rid of his shoes, shirt, and pants, to be as light as possible in the water.

We begin by swimming with clothing in the shallow end, swimming across one side to the other side (so swim across lane one to nine or however many lanes there are). This will build muscle and endurance, and he gets used to what's happening as this is a change of environment.

It will be difficult with clothing, however, your buoyancy will still be sufficient to relax and to float, which is your recovery to gain more energy or 'Resurgence'. Training with clothing on creates resistance training, which in turn builds muscle and strength.

Aston-Martin did struggle with coordination, his methods were unorthodox, however we built on his own techniques. These will be different for everyone and if they don't do the correct method, but you see that it's working and their head stays above water, just help them to perfect the technique they are using — work smarter not harder, as they say.

Using these techniques to build confidence in the water will help give you more time to get to safety or back to shore. Treading water, breath control, buoyancy, and underwater drills are the basics of water confidence. I recommend this phase be done over 5 sessions with each session going for 60 minutes in duration with breaks, or until they grasp the concept of the techniques.

2. Underwater Pool Competency: Candidates learn essential skills like *knot tying*, Advanced *buoyancy control*, and *underwater navigation*. They practise these skills while submerged in the pool.

The second part of the program would usually commence in week two, however this is dependent on the candidate's ability during the first week. If more time is required then the second week would basically be a continuation of the first week.

Here we step it up a notch, and begin learning how to tie knots under water. This will take time. You can do this standing in the water then ducking your head under water and commence tying the knot. This also helps with breath control and holding our breath. For Aston-Martin this was no more than 20 seconds, which is okay, it's not a race and we're not going for the record, it's just to get them into the frame of mind to relax in the water. Staying calm and focused and to not panic is the very essence to surviving in the water.

1st Technique: knot tying - Tying knots is not difficult, but it requires fine motor skills to learn how to tie a knot. Aston-Martin would practise this out of the water, but it was difficult for him to do, so we modified this session to have him try to tie any kind of knot or at least play with the rope's two ends and see what he made of this. Then we asked him do this under water.

The first few times he lasted about five seconds under water, as he had to train his brain to do a few different things, firstly, hold breath under water, second use both hands to control the rope under water, thirdly begin to tie a knot — or play with the rope and try to make a mess of it, which was easier. After four attempts, he began to understand what he had to do, however this would only be a short increase. It is a good exercise to learn as if you ever become stuck under water due to underwater debris and your shoelace gets caught, instead of panicking, just relax and simply undo the lace or get rid of the shoe.

2nd Technique: the advanced buoyancy control - Which is basically moving under water and at various depths to avoid debris, or if you are in a boat and it has capsized, you might have to get from one section to the other but have to go underwater due to debris or items in the boat that are now in your way.

The importance of this technique is simple. Every time you use a muscle you use oxygen, plus you need to control your buoyancy so you last longer under water and can move freely, on a full breath of air you will surface due to the amount of oxygen in your body.

Laying back in the floating position, hold your breath so you float, and take very shallow breaths. Now delete a small amount of the air from your lungs, count to 2, then hold your breath. You would have submerged a bit. Now take a deep breath, and hold your breath, now you would have increased your position to the surface. To practise this, try holding your arm out and ask the child to navigate under your arm, without touching it. Using controlled buoyancy breathing, deplete the air in your lungs, count to 3, you should have dropped slightly, and then ask the child to again swim under the arm. You have to judge the amount of air in your lungs that needs to be depleted to finish the activity. This will take several attempts to get the basics right.

By controlling the amount of oxygen, you control the depth. I explained this to Aston-Martin as best as I could. It was difficult for him to understand the idea and what to do, but we did the best we could under the circumstances. He did well and I was happy, as he understood the need to move underwater, which was a good sign that he managed to get something out of it. I recommend doing this exercise several times, and have them submerge a few centimetres under the water, and then change depth by forcing a bit of air out, swimming at a new depth, then back up to the surface. Do this until you can see they have full control of the depth using advanced buoyancy control.

3rd Technique: underwater navigation – This is fun and is more about building confidence in the pool, but you use a compass and practise navigating under water. The concept is the same as if you were out of the water. An easy exercise, it is more to build confidence, increase breath control skills, buoyancy skills, treading water skills and underwater swimming skills. So, we are basically taking what we learnt so far and putting it all together.

For Aston-Martin it was difficult as he needed to understand how the compass worked. You basically let them know that the arrow will tell them which way they are facing or wanting to go. He had never seen a compass before and never used one until this session. So, we took a bit of time to get him to visualize where to go by following the arrow and the letters which represent N, E, S, W. I asked him if you want to go and follow the N directions, where does the arrow need to point? He replied with "N". To which I said. "Yes, that is correct." Teaching them basic compass navigation will help the process.

So, I said to Aston-Martin that I wanted him to go into the water, look at the compass, then swim underwater and go to N, count to 3, then go to E and count to 2, then come up to the surface. He struggled in the beginning, but I was in the water to help him. It was a good way to get him to think — hand, eye, brain coordination — they have to think outside the box and understand how to use the compass correctly. We would continue by saying go under water, and go to S then count for 3, then go to W and count to 3, then go to E and count to 3 and then surface. He would do this quickly and get a bit confused, but he understood what he had to do, so the concept for him worked, it was just going to take more time.

We spent twenty minutes on this, and eventually he understood and went okay, it was not 100%, but he knew what he had to do. This exercise gets the brain working, but more so you are doing more things underwater with them so you are building their confidence more and more by undertaking various scenarios underwater. They are training their brain to cope with different environmental scenarios, which they will remember and use if the need ever called for it.

By the end of the second week, we have done enough sessions to build up confidence in the pool. Continuing to use these skills will only help build confidence, which is our aim, and to help with survival techniques in oceans, rivers, lakes etc.

3. Drownproofing: This exercise involves performing various techniques, such as being fully clothed and taking them off combined with buoyancy bobbing, floating and controlled breathing, all in a singular motion.

The third week we look into drownproofing. This is not difficult; the instructions are simple and easy to follow. Pools are where most people end up in trouble, and pool depth will vary, but the most common average depth pool in Australia is 1.7 metres deep, although occasionally you will have one that is 2 metres deep.

1st Technique: Clothing off – A great deal of the time the child or person will land in the water fully clothed — so the aim is to use simple techniques to get the clothing off. Start by NEVER EVER TREAD WATER FULLY CLOTHED. You burn too much energy and get tired quickly. So, start by going to the bottom and, along the way, use your toes to push the heels of your shoes until they come off. *(This is why you don't tie shoe laces tight, just enough to keep them on ☺).* Once you're at the bottom, push yourself up and get to the surface, arch your head back, and hold your breath so you float, conserving energy, then with your toes continue to push the shoes off.

2nd Technique: Buoyancy bobbing continuation – Continue to sink to the bottom, relax, and stand on the ground, bend your legs, and push yourself up, back towards the surface taking your shoes off, using your toes. Once this is done, undo your jeans/shorts slowly.

1.1 Advanced Technique – *for those that are able, if you have jeans, tie a knot at the bottom ends of the jeans together, (ankles). Close the zipper, and squeeze as much water as you can from the pants above your head. Then like the game of soccer (throw in) grab the pants by the waist and wave them over your head to fill them with air and land in the water in one single motion, squeeze the waist tight (use shoelaces if you can). Place your head through both left and right jean legs and use like a normal life vest ☺.*

3rd Technique: Undress while floating - Once the jeans and shoes are off, depending on the shirt, keep it on if it is light, if it's a heavy material shirt then take it off but keep it close to you, continue to float and slowly take the rest of the clothing off. You should have bike pants, undies or boxers on only and a light material shirt. Lean back, hold breath and float, taking shallow breaths, and conserve energy. Slowly make your way back to the side of the pool.

A 1.7 metre pool is a good depth to train a child in, as it will get them used to the depth and they know how many strokes it takes to get to the surface, and how hard they have to push from the bottom to get to the surface. So, we now understand the importance of floating. Aston-Martin is good at this and I'm comfortable that if he gets tired, he will simply lay on his back, take a deep breath and hold it, and he will be floating comfortably and can use his arms and push like a bird towards the edge of the pool.

For Aston-Martin, removing his clothes proved to be very difficult, and although we tried a few times, he was not able to complete the task. This is okay as it is not an easy task to complete. He just needs more time and we will continue to train in this area. I make sure he always wears light clothing, which is why I buy cheap shorts which are loose and are the pull-off kind with no zipper, just pull-up and pull-down type shorts. I buy his shirts at Target or Kmart, because they are light and loose and easy to take off. Jeans are more difficult, and requires more training, so I highly recommend pull-up shorts.

I made sure the techniques we did in weeks one and two were drilled into Aston-Martin, as it's important for these children to understand accidents can happen and people can accidently fall into pools, creeks, rivers or from boats into the ocean. And panicking is not going to help. So, by making sure Aston-Martin is confident in swimming pools with safety techniques is more important than learning how to swim 100 metres or 50 metres as he won't have the strength to do this. If they fall into a pool, it's about using the right technique to get to the surface and to the edge of the pool.

4. Distance Swim: Candidates practise swimming techniques and endurance drills, simulating scenarios where they may need to swim long distances in challenging conditions.

Here in week four, we use the kickboard and a life vest, either Styrofoam or air floaties. The kickboard worked, he would just have to hold the board and use his legs to kick.

1st Technique: life vest swim – Here we get them used to swimming long distances, and by distance, I mean I'm only getting Aston-Martin to swim 25 metres as for him it is about getting the technique right. Life vests are thin and easy to use and they are great when boating, but they limit you in the water, so for him it was about laying backwards and kicking while looking left and right and changing direction when required. Laying backwards conserves energy.

2nd Technique: on-off life vest swim – Every child knows how to put on a shirt or vest and how to take it off. So, the same dynamics apply here. We swim and we take off the vest and use it to float, then we go around or under an object, then return to the surface, and put the life vest back on. This is good for children who are in a lake or river or whichever scenario involves debris. You can't swim through debris. So, going under is the most logical. Unzip the vest, take it off completely and hold onto the vest. Using the buoyancy bobbing and breathing control technique, we go under a simulated piece of debris then resurface and put the vest back on.

This is more of a fun scenario, but it gets them use to understanding dangers and what to do and how to do it. Some children will have limited capabilities and may not fully understand how to do this technique. Keep it simple and use the first group of techniques we started with. This means you will need to be very careful with the child around water areas.

The extra week we did was the fifth week — where we went to the beach and I taught Aston-Martin the importance of *surf passage*. This is where we teach them how to navigate the surf as it's the most challenging of any water type. The waves are challenging, however by using the right techniques you can build yours and their confidence in the ocean and how to handle the conditions.

5. Surf Passage: Candidates train to handle rough surf conditions, including swimming through waves.

Handling rough surf conditions and swimming through waves can be daunting, but with practice and the right techniques, you can become more confident and capable. Aston-Martin enjoyed the training, it was fun and it was a great experience for him, but he quickly understood that mother nature will not be nice and is unforgiving. We used what we had learned and practised over the last four weeks and applied this to ocean swimming.

Build your swimming skills: Start by improving your overall swimming abilities. Practise different strokes, such as freestyle and breaststroke because they are the easiest. Backstroke is not a great idea if you're going into the waves as you won't see them and if you're coming into shore, you will have to stop repeatedly to self-adjust your direction and then start again, which is wasting energy. To build strength and endurance in the water training is required and starting off in a local swimming pool is best. It's important to be a strong and confident swimmer before attempting to handle rough surfing conditions. And always swim with a friend, never alone.

Learn about the waves: Understand how waves work and how they can affect your swimming. Learn about wave patterns, tides, and how waves break. This knowledge will help you anticipate and navigate through the waves more effectively. You need to remember that ocean swimming takes up a lot of energy. Aston-Martin got tired quickly, we took it slow and started at Bribie Island as the waves are small, so it was a great starting point. Going directly to the Sunshine Coast or Gold Coast beaches is nice, but remember the waves are larger and rougher so not the best. With Aston-Martin it was better to start small and aim high, and Bribie Island was the perfect place.

In the Navy you're taught everything you know about water because you are living on it. All the dangers associated with oceans, the dos and don'ts.

Here, I'm going to explain the differences between waves and potential dangers. I took Aston-Martin to Bribie Island beach and we sat on the sand and watched the waves, this is highly recommended so you can sense what is happening. I explained to Aston-Martin the types of waves, knowing he won't remember them all, and may not remember each wave and what the potential dangers are, but he would know a big wave or a small wave, plus the most important aspect of any beach are the yellow and red flags that we must swim between. He understands this well, and sees the yellow/red life guards and flags.

Various types of waves have their own characteristics and potential dangers. Here are some common types of waves:

1. **Spilling waves:** These waves are often found in milder surf conditions. They break gently and gradually, creating a white, foamy line as they roll towards the shore. Spilling waves are generally considered less dangerous and are more suitable for beginners. These are the ones at Bribie Island (hint, hint).

2. **Plunging waves:** Plunging waves are more powerful and have a steeper face compared to spilling waves. They break with a curling crest and can be exciting for experienced surfers. However, plunging waves can also be more challenging to navigate and may have strong currents near the breaking point, making them potentially more dangerous. You can get sucked back out into the ocean due to the previous wave's water going back.

3. **Surging waves:** Surging waves are characterised by a powerful and abrupt rise in water that doesn't necessarily break. They can be unpredictable and have a strong

backwash, making them hazardous for swimmers or surfers who may get caught in the turbulent water.

4. **Dumping waves:** Dumping waves are known for their intense breaking action. They break forcefully and abruptly, often with a powerful impact. Dumping waves can be very challenging to swim or surf in, as they can create strong currents and may cause injuries if not approached with caution. You will know when you see a dumping wave because it is loud.

5. **Rogue waves:** Rogue waves are exceptionally large and unexpected waves that can occur even in relatively calm conditions. They are rare, but when they occur, they can be extremely dangerous, with the potential to capsize boats or catch swimmers off-guard. You won't know until you are in one, however they are very rare.

So, after explaining these to Aston-Martin, for him to fully understand, I kept it simple: small waves are okay, big waves are not okay.

Timing is key: Timing is crucial when swimming through waves. Watch the waves and wait for a lull or a break in the wave sets before you start swimming. This will give you a better chance to make progress without being constantly pushed back by the waves. When you enter the water wait for the wave to have broken and gone past you, then commence swimming.

Dive under the waves: As a wave approaches, you can dive under it to avoid getting tossed around. Take a deep breath, push down on the water with your hands, and dive under the waves. Stay low and streamline your body to minimise resistance. You may find yourself going slightly back towards shore, this is due to the force that's behind the wave.

Maintain body position: When swimming through waves, keep your body streamlined and your head down. This will help you maintain forward momentum and reduce the chance of getting pushed back by the waves.

Use your arms and legs: Use your arms and legs to propel yourself forward through the waves. Coordinate your strokes with your kicking to generate power and maintain a steady pace. Keep your movements strong and controlled.

Stay calm and focused: It's important to stay calm and focused when swimming through waves. If you get caught in a wave or knocked off balance, try to stay relaxed and regain your composure. Panic can make it more difficult to navigate through the surf.

Practise in controlled environments: Start practising in controlled environments, such as a swimming pool with wave machines or a calm beach with small waves. Dreamworld's 'White water world' has small waves so this is a great place to start. Gradually progress to more challenging conditions as you gain confidence and experience. At Bribie Island the waves were small and were spilling waves. Aston-Martin did okay, he needed to build his strength, but he was confident in the water and that's important. He did not panic and did not fear the waves, he kept going until he got good at the technique.

The next important talk we had about the ocean was what we call 'The RIP'. So here is an easy explanation which you can tell your child, this is how I explained it to Aston-Martin.

The RIP, also known as a *rip current*, is a powerful flow of water that moves away from the shore and out into the ocean. Imagine you're at the beach, and you see the waves crashing onto the shore. Sometimes, in between those crashing waves, there's a special kind of current called a rip current. It's like a fast and sneaky river that flows from the beach back into the ocean.

Here's how it happens: When big waves come to the shore, they bring lots of water with them. But sometimes, that water needs to go back out to the open ocean. So, it finds a way to escape by making a rip current. It's like a secret tunnel underwater!

Now, rip currents can be a bit tricky because they're strong and can pull you away from the shore. But don't worry, there are things we can do to stay safe:

1. **Spotting a rip current:** Look for areas where the waves don't seem to be breaking like the others. It might look like a calm or foamy path of water that's moving away from the beach.
2. **Stay away from it:** If you see a rip current, it's important not to swim or play in that area. The current can be very powerful and make it hard to swim back to the shore.
3. **Stay calm and call for help:** If you accidentally get caught in a rip current, it's essential to stay calm and not panic. Remember, it won't pull you under the water, but it can take you away from the shore. Signal for help by waving your arms and calling for a lifeguard or an adult nearby. But remember week one, when we spoke about buoyancy and floating and holding your breath, this is what you do, so you're not using up energy. Let the rip take you out.
4. **Float and go with the flow:** If you're caught in a rip current and can't swim back to the shore, try to float on your back or tread water. The current will eventually stop pulling you out, and **then you can swim parallel to the shore, which means swimming sideways along the beach**. This will help you escape the current and get back to safety.

Remember, rip currents are a natural part of the ocean, and it's important to always swim with adult supervision and follow the instructions of lifeguards. By being aware and knowing what to do, we can enjoy the beach while staying safe from rip currents. Always swim between the yellow and red flags with lifeguards. Every time Aston-Martin sees the beach and the yellow and red flags, he remembers lifeguards, and swimming between those flags. This is part of his long-term memory, but this took several years to become part of his long-term memory.

An example of what a boot camp would look like is listed for you below, which you can use if you wish. The course is a four-week course, however, I would condense this into two weeks and just take the important aspects into consideration. I would look at your child's strengths and weaknesses and build on these.

Aston-Martin's school holidays are structured differently, and I take my time to implement a strict routine and structure for him, to achieve life skills. I would cram what I would normally want to do in four weeks into two weeks as his school holidays were only two weeks long. I use the activities that Aston-Martin likes, and the ones he does not want to do we simply don't do. Some days he does not want to spend the whole day there, which is okay. The initial idea was to create an entire day's worth of activities and then go based on his mood and capabilities. We may not always get through every one, and this is fine. They may prefer to play more, so incorporating the activities into their play would be a good idea; don't push if they don't want to, just ease into it.

Week 1:

8:30 am - 9:00 am:	Warm-up exercises (gentle stretching, light cardio)
9:00 am - 9:45 am:	Walking session (focus on building endurance)
9:45 am - 10:00 am:	Drink break
10:00 am - 10:30 am:	Swimming techniques (introduction to treading water)
10:30 am - 11:00 am:	Snack break
11:00 am - 11:45 am:	Water Fitness session (low-impact exercises, body resistance movements)
11:45 am - 12:30 pm:	Lunch break
12:30 pm - 1:30 pm:	Memory activity (Face me, throw objects in water behind him, and he needs to locate them using memory, sensory, and sound)

1:30 pm - 2:15 pm:	Rest and relaxation (quiet activities, mindfulness exercises)
2:15 pm - 3:00 pm:	Drink break and swimming techniques (duck diving)
3:00 pm - 4:00 pm:	Water resistance training (walking in water, free movement, underwater swimming drills)
4:00 pm - 4:15 pm:	Snack break
4:15 pm - 5:00 pm:	Cool-down exercises and stretching.
5:00 pm:	End of the day

Weeks 2-4:

The following weeks can consist of similar activities, but with gradual progression and variations to keep the participants engaged and motivated. Here are some ideas:

1. Increase the duration and intensity of walking, jogging, and running sessions gradually over time.
2. Introduce more advanced swimming techniques, such as tying rope underwater and specific underwater techniques.
3. Incorporate ankle weight techniques into strength training exercises but start with very light weights and progress cautiously.
4. Include fun and challenging obstacle courses or circuit training to keep the activities diverse and exciting.
5. Offer educational sessions on nutrition and healthy eating habits during snack or lunch breaks.

Remember to always prioritise the safety and wellbeing of the participants, providing modifications and alternatives for those with physical limitations. It's also important to consult with medical professionals or specialists familiar with Prader-Willi Syndrome to ensure the activities are appropriate for the participants.

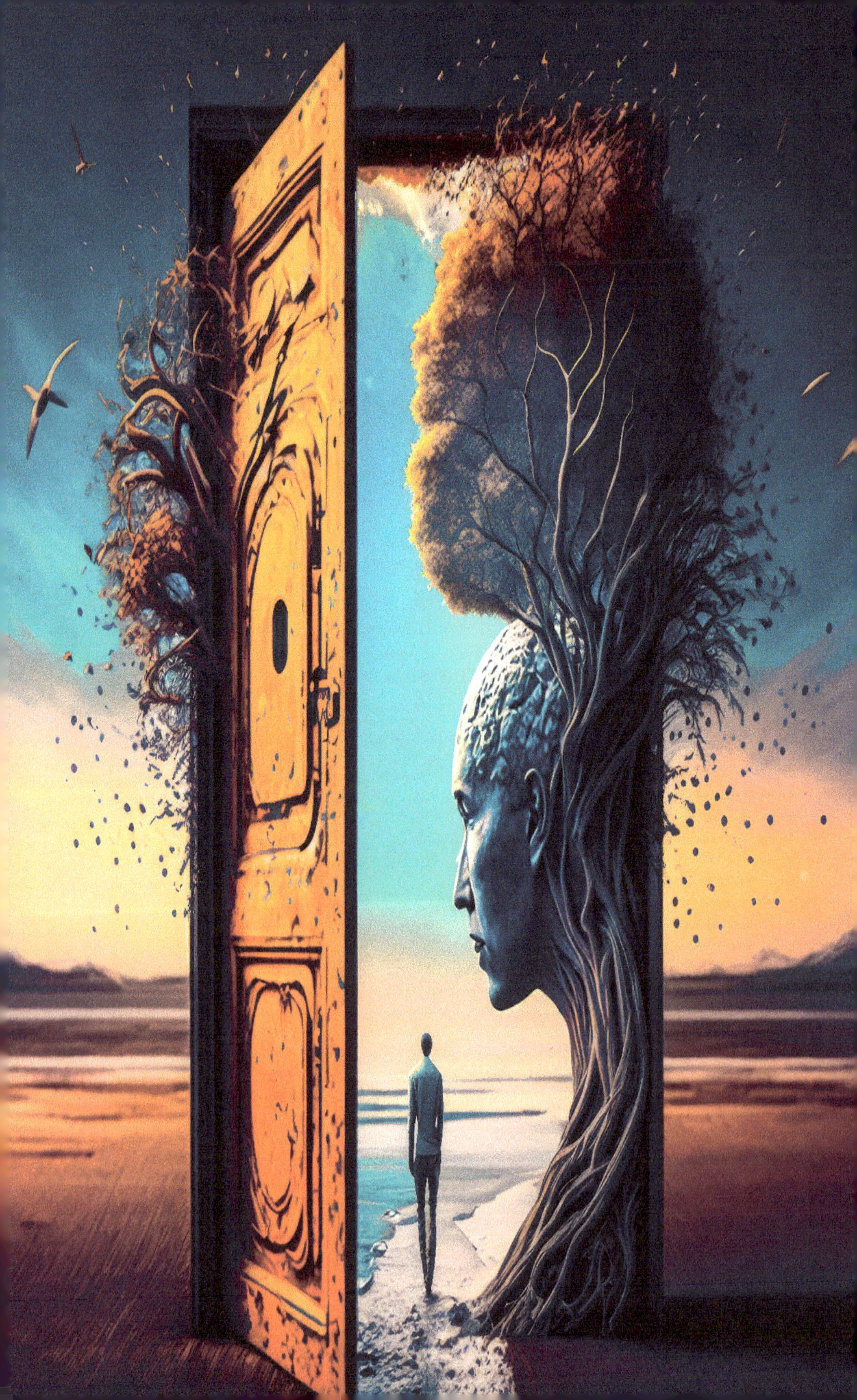

CHAPTER 19

Understanding Behavioural Problems & the Six Levels of Disquietude

Prader-Willi Syndrome (PWS) is named after the two Swiss doctors who first described it in 1956, Andrea Prader and Heinrich Willi. This syndrome is characterised by a variety of physical, cognitive, and behavioural challenges. While the physical symptoms of PWS are well-documented, its associated behavioural problems often pose significant challenges for individuals with the syndrome and their families. In this chapter, we will explore the behavioural problems which I have commonly observed and the underlying causes, and potential strategies for managing these challenges which have helped through early intervention.

First and foremost, it is imperative to recognise that the behavioural manifestations in Prader-Willi Syndrome diverge from those observed in other syndromes, and the variability in these behaviours among affected children necessitates tailored treatment and management approaches. Drawing from insights gleaned from specialists, medical literature, research endeavours focusing on PWS, and the experiences of other parents of individuals with PWS, along with the implementation of personalised management programs, I have amassed a comprehensive understanding of this complex condition.

Throughout my tenure of observation and research, certain consistent behavioural patterns have come to the fore. Behavioural outbursts often stem from the repetition of queries, particularly the persistent reiteration of "how" for every answer you provide. I observed that responses to a "how" question from a PWS child can trigger an outburst due to their difficulty in understanding the answer/s. It becomes apparent that the response of "how" does not align with the majority of the provided answers, making it progressively more challenging to answer the "how". Thus, while the repetition may seem superfluous to the observer, it signifies a genuine lack of comprehension on the part of the individual with PWS, necessitating alternative modes of explanation. This recurrent pattern is indicative of underlying speech and language challenges, contributing to the individual's difficulty in grasping the intended meaning of communicated words.

Similarly, the incessant repetition of "why" following a comprehensive explanation engenders heightened emotional distress, potentially escalating into temper outbursts when met with repetitive responses or variations thereof from the caregiver.

A spectrum of observable indicators encompassing lying on the ground, stomping of feet, door slamming, kicking, object throwing, destructive tendencies, crying, yelling, and exhibiting angry facial expressions have been documented.

These observations delineate a sequential progression of perturbed emotional states observed in certain individuals grappling with Prader-Willi Syndrome.

Based on my extensive longitudinal observations, I have deduced the existence of a hierarchical taxonomy of emotional perturbation in individuals afflicted with Prader-Willi Syndrome. This taxonomy delineates six discrete levels of disquietude, numbered sequentially from one to six.

1. **Incipient reactivity:** Characterised by elevated vocalizations, often inquiries seeking clarification or elaboration upon a directive or topic of discussion, slight jumping (podal movement) occurs. Signs of unease such as fidgeting or mild agitation with the environmental stimuli or social situation
2. **Mild provocation:** Evidenced by mild kinetic behaviours such as minor podal movements delivered at an increased cadence or intensity when seeking understanding. Escalating vocal protests may accompany if comprehension remains elusive. Verbal expressions of discomfort include statements of dissatisfaction or disengagement. Tone of voice may become more pronounced.
3. **Moderate agitation:** Typified by rapidly shifting facial expressions conveying mounting agitation or frustration. Kinaesthetic movements concurrently accelerate alongside intensifying vocalizations, rapid podal movement and self-hitting. Physical manifestations of restlessness like pacing or fiddling emerge. Compliance with directives starts to wane.
4. **Intermittent disquietude:** Marked by auto affective or self-directed actions likely emanating from a lack of directive comprehension or recollection. Attempts at independent sense-making emerge. Throwing of objects. Outward shows of distress intensify through actions including stomping, door slamming or crying. Emotional deregulation becomes apparent.
5. **Advanced turbulence:** Wherein both verbal and non-verbal communications become coarser, more illogical and potentially threatening in nature, signalling an exacerbated state by throwing object towards person(s). Potentially harmful behaviours may arise presenting a risk of injury. Throwing objects, kicking or hitting may transpire. Complete lack of behavioural control.

6. **Profound perturbation:** When physical conduct abruptly escalates, potentially endangering oneself or others through intentional psychomotor actions. Concomitant property damage also poses a risk at this stage due to degraded control of impulses. Maximum escalation occurs, characterised by unmitigated emotional tempest and danger to self or others. Violent conduct is plausible, demanding immediate specialist intervention.

This graded scale of the disquietude phenomenon aids systematic comprehension and customised support for de-escalation at each phase before full blown behavioural crises ensue.

Diffusing the six levels of disquietude

Level 1 to 2 you can quickly diffuse given the right tools to do this. It's imperative to *whisper* when you communicate to avoid the situation getting out of hand and increasing to the next level. The reason you whisper is that some people with PWS are sensitive to loud noises or have sensory issues, which can make them feel anxious, stressed, or overwhelmed by certain sounds or environments. If you yell or scream with facial expressions, this will increase their anxiety, and thus increases the levels of aggression. Also, don't say 'No', as this word does not sit well with them. Substitute the word 'No', with 'Let's both have a look at this together'. Sounds more promising, and defuses the situation to the point where they will acknowledge that you are engaged with their issue.

It's very important to note that if you decide to go against them head on, by yelling or screaming back, this will only accelerate the levels more quickly. Remember, their chromosome condition is not their fault, they are not able to regulate emotions. We can control our emotions, whereas they can't. So, what I do is I speak softly and introduce one of their favourite toys, teddy bears or places they like. This is an example of what I would say when it gets to level 1 or 2.

"Hey Aston-Martin, I spoke with Rexy today, and he was wanting to know if you want to go on a train ride today".

Or *"Hey Aston-Martin, I spoke with Rexy just before and he wants to go to the kid's park as there are children that will most likely be there and want to play. Did you want to go with Rexy"* (use a favourite toy/teddy).

You need to play it simple and keep calm. You need to show patience first and foremost — which could be difficult for most people, as your limits will be pushed. Having backup plans/ideas will help you, such as daily outdoor events are always good even if it's a walk to the park or going for drive to the park. Getting them out of the house environment will help.

Using a continuous, calm, soothing voice will help bring them down to your level. The main problem is they will not fully understand, which means you will need to explain this in a different way, and sometimes in multiple different ways. It's best to understand the characteristics first and try to remember them, so you are prepared.

What IF we reach level 6?

Well, in this case, it's not your fault, and not their fault. Here is what I do when we get to level 6. I quickly bring in his dinosaur Rexy, and I hug Aston-Martin, and whisper into his ear that Rexy wants to make a healthy cupcake. As he likes to make food, we can orchestrate a healthy option to make a healthy sweet. This idea brought down his level almost instantly, and we both ventured into the kitchen and we made cupcakes. I use *Lakanto No Added Sugar Vanilla Cupcake Mix 360g*, it's a healthier option as it is *98% sugar free, 40% lower carbs, 36% Less Calories*. I let Aston-Martin make the cupcakes, and help him with this. I don't always do the food routine, however if you keep it simple and healthy then this is okay, so next time you can make a healthy shake, or dinner, so you have options.

I noted that with Aston-Martin, when I whisper this into his ear, he quickly de-stresses and his anxiety level reduces almost instantly. He then has a small burst of laughing, crying, smiling, and when this happens, he wants to know more, so you quickly explain what it is you're going to do. Ideally, you want to give a few options for them, so park, cupcake or bubbles would be sufficient, and he gets to choose what he wants to do with Rexy. It works, but you need to have backup plans, creating an imaginative world does work.

Chapter 19.1

Techniques for Parents

Let me share with you some of the most useful techniques that I found were effective with Aston-Martin. Most of these have been mentioned before, and are summarised below for ready reference.

Effective Communication Techniques

Active Listening: Practise active listening by giving your full attention to your child when they are speaking. Maintain eye contact, nod, and provide verbal cues to show that you are engaged and understanding them. Being engaged directly with eye contact shows them you're listening, which is what they want. If you disengage, this shows them you are not interested, and this is when they begin to become upset and the onset of behavioural issues slowly start to climb.

Use Clear and Simple Language: Adapt your communication style to match your child's understanding level. Use clear and simple language, break down complex instructions into small steps, and use visual aids or gestures to support your communication. They won't understand some words, and to them this is frustrating — to the magnitude of if we were in an interview and I threw in the word *sesquipedalian* and I asked you to use it in a sentence and you had ten seconds to make the sentence and if you succeed you get the job.

Visual Supports: Use visual supports, such as picture schedules, social stories or visual cues to help your child understand and follow routines, expectations, and rules.

Choice Offering: Provide choices to your child whenever possible to give them a sense of control and promote their independence. For example, offer options like "Would you like to wear the red shirt or the blue shirt today?"

Positive Behaviour Management Strategies

Reinforcement: Use positive reinforcement techniques, such as praise, rewards or tokens to acknowledge and encourage your child's appropriate behaviour. This can motivate them to repeat desired behaviours. Don't combine food with rewards unless it's a very healthy food, but best to not associate food and rewards.

Behaviour Contracts: Develop behaviour contracts with your child, setting clear expectations and rewards for meeting specific goals or exhibiting desired behaviours. This helps create a sense of accountability and provides structure.

Visual Cues and Reminders: Use visual cues or reminders, such as a behaviour chart or a visual timer, to help your child understand expectations, track progress, and manage their time effectively.

Structured Routine: Establish a structured routine with predictable schedules and clear transitions. This can help reduce anxiety and provide a sense of security and stability for your child.

Stress Management Skills

Self-Care: Take care of yourself as a parent, ensuring you have time for rest, relaxation and personal activities. This helps you manage your own stress levels, enabling you to better support your child. Listen to 'Space ambient music', it's best to consider instrumental music or genres like classical music without lyrics as this is less distracting.

Deep Breathing and Relaxation Techniques: Teach your child deep breathing exercises and relaxation techniques to help them manage stress and anxiety. Practise these techniques together in calm moments and encourage their use during challenging situations.

Sensory Regulation: Identify and understand your child's sensory sensitivities and provide appropriate strategies to help them regulate their sensory experiences. This may include using sensory tools like fidget toys, rice in a bucket with a toy buried, providing sensory breaks, or creating a calm sensory environment.

Every child is unique

It is important to note that every child is unique, and what works for one child may not work for another. It is recommended you consult with professionals, such as therapists or behaviour specialists, who can provide personalised guidance and strategies tailored to your child's specific needs. Also, just for your information: 'The professor's lectures were filled with sesquipedalian language, leaving the students perplexed and reaching for their dictionaries'. Now you know!

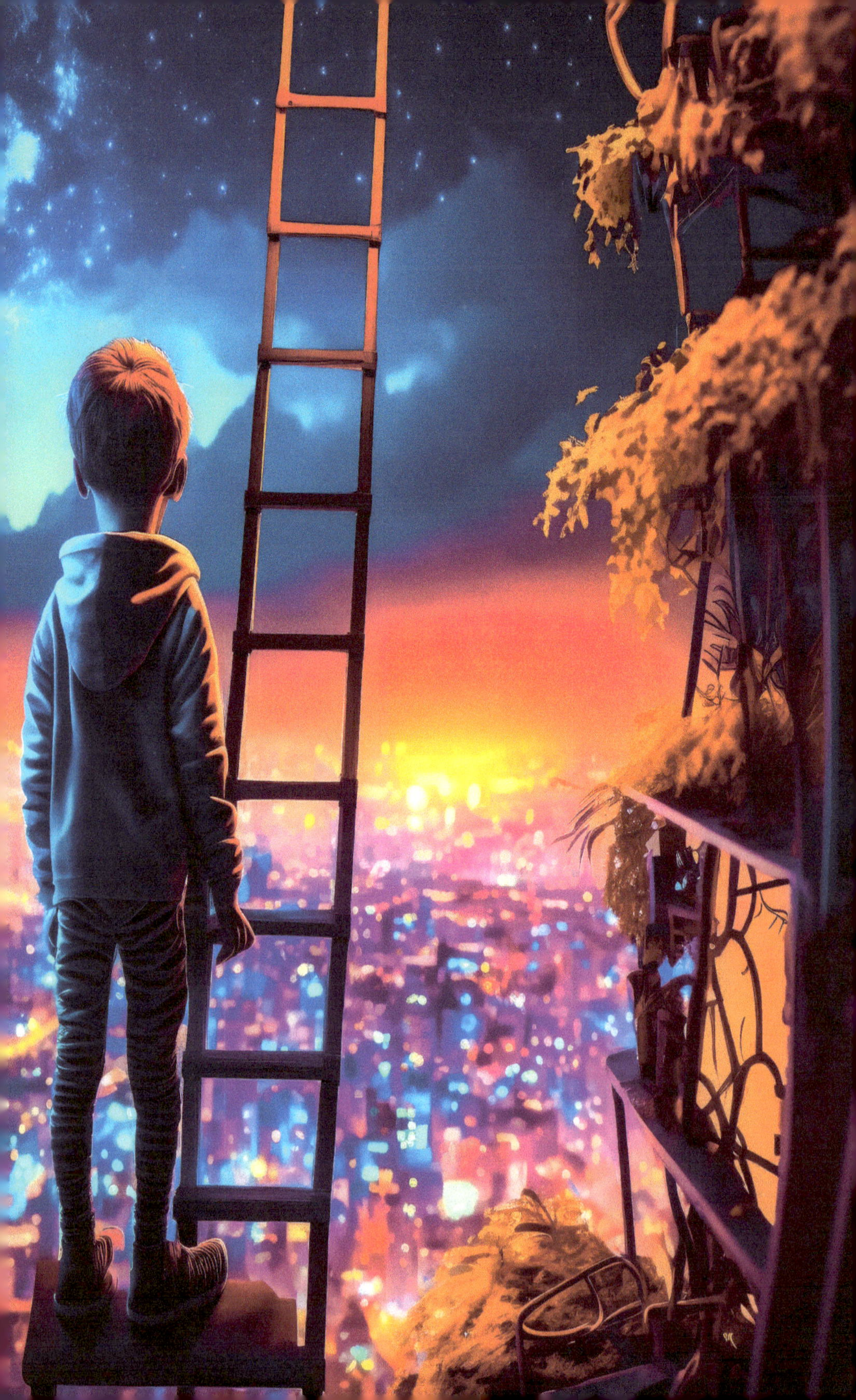

Chapter 20

The Sequential Positive Behaviour Management Program

Aston-Martin is the first participant to engage in a specialised program from home — which I designed based on him and his PWS characteristics. The program is the *Sequential Positive Behaviour Management Program*. This program focuses on a structured daily routine and is based on a 'coach-athlete relationship', by implementing parental influences for special needs children. I aim to incorporate a motivational model and introduce autonomous positive supportive behaviour.

Coach-Athlete relationship

The 'coach-athlete relationship' is a concept commonly used in the field of sports psychology to describe the dynamic interaction between a coach and an athlete. It encompasses the various ways in which the coach influences the athlete's motivation, performance and overall development. In this relationship, the coach plays a pivotal role in providing guidance, support and expertise to the athlete. They are responsible for teaching the athlete essential skills, techniques and strategies relevant to their sport. The coach also offers feedback, constructive criticism and encouragement to help the athlete improve their performance.

However, the 'coach-athlete relationship' is not solely about the coach motivating the athlete. It also recognises the importance of the athlete's own self-motivation and drive to excel. While the coach can provide external motivation through their guidance and support, it is ultimately up to the athlete to cultivate their internal motivation and commitment to achieve their goals. The coach's role in fostering motivation is multifaceted. They can create a positive and supportive training environment that encourages the athlete's autonomy, competence and relatedness. By providing opportunities for the athlete to make choices and have a sense of control over their training, the coach helps to enhance the athlete's intrinsic motivation. Moreover, the coach can help the athlete set meaningful and challenging goals, breaking them down into smaller achievable targets. This goal-setting process can enhance the athlete's motivation by providing them with a clear direction and a sense of progress. The coach-athlete relationship also involves effective communication and trust.

The coach should strive to establish open lines of communication, actively listen to the athlete's concerns, and provide constructive feedback. This supportive communication fosters a sense of trust and mutual understanding, which contributes to the athlete's motivation and willingness to work towards their goals. While the coach's primary role is to provide skills, techniques, and some motivation, the 'coach-athlete relationship' recognises that the athlete's self-motivation is crucial for sustained success. The athlete must take ownership of their training, set personal goals, and cultivate a strong work ethic. Ultimately, the coach and athlete work together in a collaborative partnership, with the coach providing guidance and support while the athlete takes responsibility for their own motivation and performance.

It is essential to comprehend that the child in question has a genetic abnormality or condition involving chromosomes. In simple terms, in your role as a coach here, you need to recognise the limitations of an athlete with PWS or any other genetic abnormality, understand the limitations, and prepare strategies to counter them.

CHAPTER 20.1

The five steps

The five steps I introduced into the program to help set the scene are:

Step 1 - Instituting - house rules, structure and consistent sequences

Instituting house rules, structure and consistent sequences is of paramount importance when supporting a special needs child with behavioural issues. These measures help establish a routine that aids in memory retention, particularly for children with short-term memory difficulties. For instance, in the case of Aston-Martin, it is crucial to provide him with a structured environment. Even though he may inquire about the day's activities upon returning from his special school, it is essential we maintain consistency in the daily routine. Aston-Martin's cognitive limitations prevent him from attending mainstream school and comprehending subjects like math, science, and English. Consequently, it is imperative for parents to be aware of their child's strengths and weaknesses, understanding what they can and cannot accomplish.

Drawing inspiration from the structured systems employed during my time in the Royal Australian Navy, I decided to incorporate a similar approach to Aston-Martin's daily chores and tasks. The most crucial aspects of recruit school were punctuality and adherence to designated locations. Being late or absent would result in stern reprimands from instructors.

By implementing a simple routine for Aston-Martin, comprising fourteen tasks (such as dressing, brushing teeth, make his bed) to be completed before catching the school bus, I then granted him the autonomy to complete them in any order. This approach fostered his sense of dependency and routine. The objective was to establish consistent sequences, enabling Aston-Martin to develop a self-regulating routine, albeit over an extended period of practice.

Throughout the seven-month duration of Aston-Martin's engagement with this daily routine, he initially encountered challenges in understanding and adapting to the tasks. I had to deploy numerous prompts to redirect his attention back to the designated tasks. Employing various strategies, one successful method involved incorporating a game-like theme, such as a chasing game or involving his favourite dinosaur toy, 'Rexy.'

By engaging in conversation with Rexy, I would inquire whether the dinosaur could assist Aston-Martin with his tasks. Aston-Martin would also participate in feeding Rexy during breakfast, although the dinosaur's food would inevitably find its way into Aston-Martin's mouth. To mitigate this, I would reduce Aston-Martin's breakfast portion and provide a separate plate with a small amount of food for Rexy. This approach was effective and enjoyable for Aston-Martin, although its efficacy diminished after a few months. Subsequently, a new game feature, such as the 'bandit' from his preferred Kids YouTube channel, was introduced. Additionally, a prize system was implemented upon completion of all tasks. It is vital to note that you will need to adapt constantly, as children gradually familiarise with and acclimate to the strategies employed, and then it doesn't work. By incorporating items of interest to the child, such as trains, and mentioning the prospect of a train ride during the task routine, a goal is established. This tactic serves as a small-scale strategy, which will be explored further in step 5.

It is best that you only offer a prize when the child is exhibiting positive behaviour and successfully completing their tasks. Associating prizes with negative behaviours or tantrums may result in the child linking the two and make it challenging for you to dissociate them. In situations where behavioural issues escalate, it may become necessary to utilize this strategy as a last resort.

However, it is advisable to explore the child's interests, such as trains, garbage trucks or dinosaurs, and communicate discreetly by whispering suggestions like, "Would you like to see a dinosaur at the museum or observe the garbage truck at the refuse tip?" Alternatively, "Would you prefer to go on a train ride?" These options provide alternative outlets if the child is exhibiting heightened behavioural episodes.

In instances where Aston-Martin's behaviour escalates, I found that a quick whisper in his ear, conveying Rexy's desire to play a game at the park, could effectively redirect his attention. By associating the visual aspect of the dinosaur toy, Rexy, with the park's enticing features like slides, sandpits and swings, his behaviour could be swiftly modified. It is crucial to sustain the imaginative world created and physically transport the child to the location outside such as a park, or your back yard, engaging in playful role-playing scenarios. The creation of an imaginary world, even if it requires leaving the house to catch an imaginary train, significantly aids in managing behavioural challenges.

In conclusion, the implementation of house rules, structure, and consistent sequences is really useful when you are supporting a special needs child with behavioural issues. By establishing routines and adhering to them consistently, parents can assist their child in developing memory retention and a sense of structure. By employing these techniques, parents can effectively create a more harmonious environment for both them and their special needs children.

Step 2 - Understanding - when to offer specific praise for appropriate behaviours

Offering praise for appropriate behaviour is a valuable mechanism, but it must be consistent and sequential. When you praise your child for a specific task, it is best to consistently acknowledge their accomplishments each time they complete them. Through this repetition, they will internalise the acceptability of their actions, not only at home but also in the broader community.

Equally important is knowing when to choose your battles. Engaging in a competition with your child, where the odds of success are slim, serves no purpose. For instance, if Aston-Martin decides to engage in a "non-requested-task," such as playing with a set of Crayola Twistable Crayons - Pack of 12, he may become fixated on twisting and untwisting all twelve crayons. Considering his ADHD, which may or may not be related to Prader-Willi Syndrome, he will prioritise completing this task and employ any means necessary to do so. As a helpful tip, these crayons can be a useful tool to keep them occupied, as the twisting motion captivates their attention. To navigate this situation effectively, incorporate it into their routine within a specific timeframe. I discreetly whisper to Aston-Martin, "Hey buddy, once you finish playing with the twisty pens in five minutes, you'll need to have a shower and get ready for school, alright?" This approach maintains his equilibrium, and he complies. Once the task is completed, he proceeds upstairs to take a shower.

Avoid confrontation, such as by attempting to forcibly take away the pens or items, as this will rapidly escalate the situation, potentially leading to a regression in behaviour. However, it is important to acknowledge that there may be instances where this strategy fails, and the situation escalates despite your efforts. In such cases, an alternative approach could be to leverage a different interest, in my case, for example, Aston-Martin's interest in trains. Whispering into his ear, I might say, "Hey, do you want to go to the train station and watch some trains after school?" Given his fondness for trains, he immediately responds and his agitation subsides, allowing for easier management of his behaviour. At this point, the remaining tasks can be completed gradually, and I can then provide specific praise for his good behaviour.

It is best never to reward or offer prizes when the child is in an unhappy behavioural state. This may inadvertently reinforce the association between behavioural issues and obtaining rewards. This is how they perceive it, and it is challenging for them to unlearn this connection. Therefore, when the situation escalates, refrain from offering rewards and instead propose engaging activities, contingent upon their adherence to instructions. Under no circumstances should food be used as a reward. Associating bad behaviour with food creates an unhealthy connection.

It is important to note that yelling or raising one's voice may exacerbate the child's anxiety and stress due to potential noise sensitivity and sensory issues, leading to verbal and physical altercations. As a parent, you possess a deep understanding of your child, and drawing from your own childhood experiences may provide valuable insights into what might work for them.

Step 3 - Applying - repetition activities, developmentally appropriate directions and commands

When providing directions to a child with Prader-Willi Syndrome at various ages, it is important to consider their unique developmental challenges. Individuals with PWS often experience what is known as "Global developmental delay", meaning their cognitive abilities may be several years behind their chronological age. For instance, a nine-year-old child **without** PWS can easily understand and follow instructions like, "Can you please go to the shed and retrieve the toolbox?" They comprehend the concept of a toolbox and can visualise it accordingly.

However, when presenting the same instruction to a nine-year-old child **with** PWS, you will need to adjust your language and approach as their mental capacity may resemble that of a much younger child. This is the case for Aston-Martin, a ten-year-old boy with PWS who exhibits a cognitive mindset similar to that of a four- or five-year-old child. Aston-Martin tends to engage better with peers of this age group at the playground, as they share similar language skills, making communication easier.

For a ten-year-old child with PWS, whose language skills may be more advanced and complex, it is best to simplify instructions and use lexically less dense words. Alternatively, one may need to break down the instruction into basic components. In some cases, continuous prompting or physically demonstrating the desired action, such as going into the shed and retrieving the toolbox, may be necessary for the child to understand the task at hand. This helps them associate words like "shed," "toolbox," and "bring" with the corresponding actions, facilitating comprehension. It is important to note that consistent prompting may still be required for future instances.

In summary, when providing directions and commands to individuals with PWS, it is necessary to consider their developmental delays and to adjust your language and the complexity of your instructions to match their cognitive abilities. Utilizing prompts, demonstrations, and imaginative distractions can effectively redirect their attention and facilitate comprehension. By employing developmentally appropriate activities and repetitive reinforcement, individuals with PWS can engage in a more positive and constructive manner, enhancing their overall communication and interaction skills.

Step 4 - Designing ahead

This is where we design in our heads where we are going, how it went last time we were there, what happened, how can we do it better, when is it safer to go. Designing ahead plays a crucial role in navigating the challenges associated with Prader-Willi Syndrome in children. Adequate planning helps to ensure successful outcomes and prevent potential issues. For instance, when taking Aston-Martin to a park, I consider factors such as the proximity to main roads and his tendency to run. Conducting a preliminary visit or using tools like Google Maps' Street view helps me to assess the suitability of a location. Regular visits to the local park provide Aston-Martin with physical exercise and social interaction.

Unfortunately, we have to avoid certain parks due to the presence of familiar children who make communication difficult for Aston-Martin, resulting in experiences of Rejection Sensitive Dysphoria (RSD). RSD, often associated with ADHD, stems from differences in brain structure, leading to heightened emotional responses to rejection. To ensure Aston-Martin's enjoyment and avoid distress for him, I carefully select suitable environments.

Visiting theme parks during non-peak times, such as weekends, offers advantages like fewer crowds and increased learning opportunities for Aston-Martin to understand community expectations. By exposing him to public spaces, he can learn about rules, identify staff members, recognise safe areas, and avoid interacting with unfamiliar individuals. Aston-Martin's one-track mind can pose risks as he may be oblivious to potential dangers while pursuing a specific goal or object, increasing the likelihood of injuries. For instance, at Dreamworld's White-Water World, he nearly ended up on a conveyor belt when attempting to move a yellow boat onto the railing system. Thankfully, timely intervention prevented a serious accident. Consequently, visiting locations beforehand and assessing the environment becomes crucial, as different settings yield different outcomes. The Gold

Coast theme parks, for example, provide a fun and enjoyable experience for Aston-Martin, fostering relaxation and a calm demeanour. However, if a desired ride is closed for maintenance, he may become upset.

I found it was essential for me to understand Aston-Martin's difficulty grasping the interconnectedness of the park and his preference for retracing steps back to the entrance. I found that demonstrating alternative routes on a map and explaining different paths within the park can assist him, although this approach may not always be effective. Riding the Dreamworld Express train and exploring the entire park on foot helped him become familiar with different sections of the park and to eventually understand that starting from the entrance for every exhibit is unnecessary.

Novel environments, unfamiliar to Aston-Martin, can trigger anxiety as he relies on familiar routes and lacks awareness of alternative paths. As Aston-Martin is visually oriented and comprehends symbols well, I found that incorporating the signage throughout Dreamworld Park and indicating our current location as well as displaying ride symbols on maps could greatly assist him. The provided park map, although challenging for Aston-Martin to interpret due to his inability to read, can serve as a reference point when combined with repeated train rides and comprehensive walks around the park. I found that repetitive reinforcement of tactics was crucial to facilitate long-term memory formation, as Aston-Martin's short-term memory poses limitations.

In summary, designing a visit ahead is a vital aspect of managing the challenges associated with PWS in children. Careful planning can help prevent issues, especially when combined with understanding your child's communication barriers, preferences, and potential emotional responses. Ultimately, a proactive approach to planning and understanding your child's unique needs is essential in ensuring their safety, wellbeing, and enjoyment in various settings.

Step 5 - Employing consistent and effective disciplinary tactics

The key word here is '**tactics**', not strategies. To me, the difference between these two words is:

a. **Strategy** – is a long-term plan which one executes step by step to achieve a goal.
b. **Tactics** – are small steps or concrete actions which one takes to achieve smaller goals to complete an action. (A good tactic has a clear purpose that aids in your strategy).

Implementing consistent and effective disciplinary tactics, with emphasis on the term 'tactics' rather than strategies, is crucial in supporting individuals with Prader-Willi Syndrome and teaching them life skills necessary for their future. The road is not a straightforward one, as it presents various challenges and detours. For instance, Aston-Martin, due to his condition, cannot thrive in a mainstream school setting where traditional subjects like math, science, religion, chemistry, and technology are taught. Therefore, he attends a special school that focuses on life skills, recognising that these skills are essential for navigating through life successfully.

To achieve success in teaching life skills to individuals with PWS, it is best to employ small, simple tactics, which serve as the building blocks that eventually form a larger strategy to accomplish the specific objectives. Repetition plays a vital role in this process, as individuals with PWS often struggle with short-term memory issues. Consistent deployment of these tactics enables them to eventually perform tasks independently, even if they may sometimes require additional support or prompting. Keep in mind that individuals with PWS tend to perceive the world in black and white with a limited tolerance for ambiguity. They rely heavily on routines and find it challenging to cope with changes.

It is important to note that individuals with PWS may engage in plausible lying, confabulation, and exaggeration as a means of manipulation. For instance, when asked if they have brushed their teeth, they may falsely claim they have in order to avoid completing the task. If confronted, individuals with PWS may vehemently insist on the truth of their statements, as they view this as an escape from fulfilling a responsibility. If met with a negative response, such as, "No, you haven't," they may persistently request a positive answer, testing the boundaries of compliance. However, by integrating toys into these activities and consistently providing clear explanations with visual aids, children are more likely to understand and cooperate, reducing their anxieties and manipulative behaviours.

Regarding Aston-Martin's daily morning and afternoon tasks, employing small tactics can facilitate his compliance. For instance, using his toy dinosaur, he is encouraged to brush Rexy's teeth while simultaneously brushing his own teeth. This simple tactic gradually transforms into a strategy, as the introduction of his beloved dinosaur motivates him to participate in the task consistently. This approach has significantly reduced instances of falsehoods regarding tooth brushing. By incorporating his favourite toy into the activity, an imaginary story is created daily, acknowledging the importance of visualising tasks in a concrete and straightforward manner.

Teaching life skills to individuals with special needs, particularly those with PWS, presents unique challenges. However, several strategies can be employed to enhance their learning experience.

CHAPTER 20.2

More useful tips

The following tips may also prove useful:

Tailor tasks to the individual's abilities: Using your understanding of the individual's needs, abilities, and readiness, choose appropriate tasks. Assigning tasks that are either too challenging or too easy can lead to frustration or disinterest.

Break tasks into smaller steps: Complex tasks can be overwhelming for individuals with special needs. Breaking them down into manageable steps allows for gradual progress and a sense of achievement at each stage.

Use visual supports: Visual aids such as schedules, charts, or pictorial representations can help your child to understand your messages better and hence to follow routines and instructions more effectively.

Incorporate preferred interests: Whenever possible, link activities to the individual's interests or preferences. This can increase motivation and engagement, making the learning experience more enjoyable.

Provide clear and concise instructions: Use simple language and concise instructions. Avoid overwhelming the individual with excessive information or complex explanations.

Offer positive reinforcement: Acknowledge and reward effort and progress with praise or small incentives. Positive reinforcement can motivate individuals to continue practising and mastering new skills.

Foster a supportive environment: Create a nurturing and supportive environment that encourages exploration and risk-taking. Celebrate accomplishments and provide constructive feedback to foster growth and self-confidence.

Collaborate with professionals: Seek guidance from professionals, such as therapists or educators experienced in working with individuals with special needs. They can provide valuable insights and tailored strategies for supporting the individual's specific needs.

Continued research and collaboration are necessary to further enhance our understanding of effective strategies and interventions for individuals with special needs, ensuring that they receive the necessary tools and resources to thrive and reach their full potential. With a combination of patience, empathy, and evidence-based practices, we can create a nurturing environment that empowers individuals with special needs to lead fulfilling and meaningful lives.

Case Study — Start of day routine

Aston-Martin's daily routine is designed to promote his independence and self-motivation. From the moment he wakes at 6:00 am each morning, he is familiar with the routine and the tasks that must be accomplished before he boards the school bus. Although the sequence in which the tasks are completed can be flexible, Aston-Martin knows the importance of addressing tasks as they arise.

Making his bed is the initial task as it is the easiest to accomplish. I emphasise to Aston-Martin that even on challenging days, returning to a well-made bed can provide a sense of comfort and order. Moving on to breakfast, Aston-Martin actively participates in setting the table and using metric cups to measure cereal — which helps him to understand what are appropriate portion sizes, which is essential for preventing overeating. By referring to the serving size instructions on the cereal box, I demonstrate the significance of following instructions and adhering to a structured routine. Introducing these concepts at an early age establishes a foundation for healthy eating habits and weight management.

CHAPTER 20.3

The Morning Tasks

The following sections provide a more academic overview of the Sequential Positive Behaviour Management Program's key elements, highlighting the importance of a well-structured routine and promoting independence.

The following sequence worked very well for Aston-Martin, and our mornings are now considerably easier.

Morning Tasks:

1. Upon awakening, encourage the child aged to demonstrate responsibility and orderliness by making their bed.
2. Engage the child in breakfast preparation, such as helping to use the metric cups and setting the table, which cultivates independence and basic measurement skills.
3. Teach the child how to use the table utensils effectively to promote self-sufficiency and enhance their fine motor skills.
4. After breakfast, prompt the child to place the dishes in the sink, reinforcing cleanliness and tidiness habits.
5. Emphasise personal hygiene and self-care skills through guided showering, either independently or with parental assistance.

6. Facilitate brushing teeth by using an electric toothbrush, providing instant feedback and reinforcing oral hygiene habits.
7. Guide the child is guided in how to dress themselves, mastering tasks such as buttoning shirts, putting on shorts, socks, and shoes, thus fostering independence in dressing.
8. Engage the child in colouring activities, such as tracing shapes, letters, and colouring within designated areas, which promote fine motor skills and cognitive development.
9. Teach the child through tracing the shape of letters how to write their name, enhancing their literacy skills and attention to detail.
10. Teach the child how to prepare their school bag, ensuring readiness to catch the school bus or enter the family car, fostering organisation and preparedness.
11. Introduce Sensory or Montessori books to stimulate the child's development and engage their sensory perception.
12. Consider incorporating soccer or football as a preferred sport choice, allowing the child to learn balancing techniques, kicking, trapping, passing, and ball control, promoting enjoyable physical activity.
13. Emphasizing safety, instruct the child not to open the bus door until the school bus has come to a complete stop and opened its doors.
14. If travelling by family car, remind the child to wear a seat belt before your departure, reinforcing safety practices.

We found that consistently adhering to this routine, improved Aston-Martin's life skills and gave him a heightened sense of predictability. Familiarity with the sequence of tasks reduced the need for my constant prompting, enabling our son to develop good self-awareness and to progress independently through his routine.

CHAPTER 20.4

The Afternoon Tasks

At the other end of the day, it is best to follow a prescribed afternoon routine to further promote independence.

Afternoon tasks:

1. Teach the child to remove their footwear and place their school bag in a designated area, encouraging good organisation.
2. Provide the child with a wholesome snack to replenish their energy levels and ensure they are properly hydrated.
3. Guide the child in changing their garments and depositing their school attire in the designated laundry container for subsequent cleaning.
4. Introduce the child to an activity booklet that incorporates tracing shapes, letters, and animals, emphasising precision and adherence to boundaries.
5. Participate in outdoor activities at the local park or embark on a leisurely walk: Use a small soccer ball to engage the child in skill-building endeavours, such as passing, trapping and kicking, while concurrently focusing on maintaining equilibrium during ball control.
6. Allow the child to enjoy unrestricted playtime at the children's park: Permit the child to interact with peers and

partake in suitable games and activities within a supervised and secure environment.

7. Involve the child in the meal preparation and setting the dining table, keeping the tasks assigned capability and age-appropriate.
8. Encourage the child to participate in household chores by assisting with the collection and arrangement of dishes in the sink.
9. Promote personal cleanliness by guiding the child through the process of showering and using an electric toothbrush to clean their teeth, thereby providing sensory feedback.
10. Resume colouring activities to foster focus, creativity and fine motor skills development.
11. Use the iPad for interactive sing-along songs and activities: If the child derives pleasure from using the iPad, incorporate it as a reward or incentive, employing the technique of exchange to swap the device for other enjoyable activities or items of value. Establish clear time limits for iPad usage and gradually reduce reliance on it over time.
12. Assist the child in preparing for sleep, ensuring they change into cozy sleep attire while refraining from using the iPad for at least one hour before sleep.
13. Encourage the child to participate in playtime with toys that offer sensory stimulation or continue engaging with the activity book.
14. Encourage the child to partake in sports-oriented endeavours or to engage in imaginative play, such as a chase game involving special characters or creating an entirely new imaginary world, thereby fostering creativity, social interaction, and physical activity.

Case Study — staying on routine

Occasionally, Aston-Martin may become engrossed in playing with toys or reading books, which is acceptable. However, the timing of such activities is important, considering our emphasis on maintaining a consistent routine.

If there is limited time in the morning, we gently redirect his attention from self-engagement tasks, as deviating from the routine can potentially lead to heightened levels of restlessness. I would say to Aston-Martin, *"Hey buddy, did you want to spend one minute or three minutes on this task before me move on to the next one"*. This leaves the option open for him to self-manage the task's completion, giving him an open-ended opportunity scenario.

It is noteworthy that the routine I devised for Aston-Martin is attuned to time management. While flexibility is permitted within the routine, adhering to a structured schedule imparts a sense of order and predictability. By instilling these principles early on, Aston-Martin has learned the value of time management and the advantages of adhering to a structured routine.

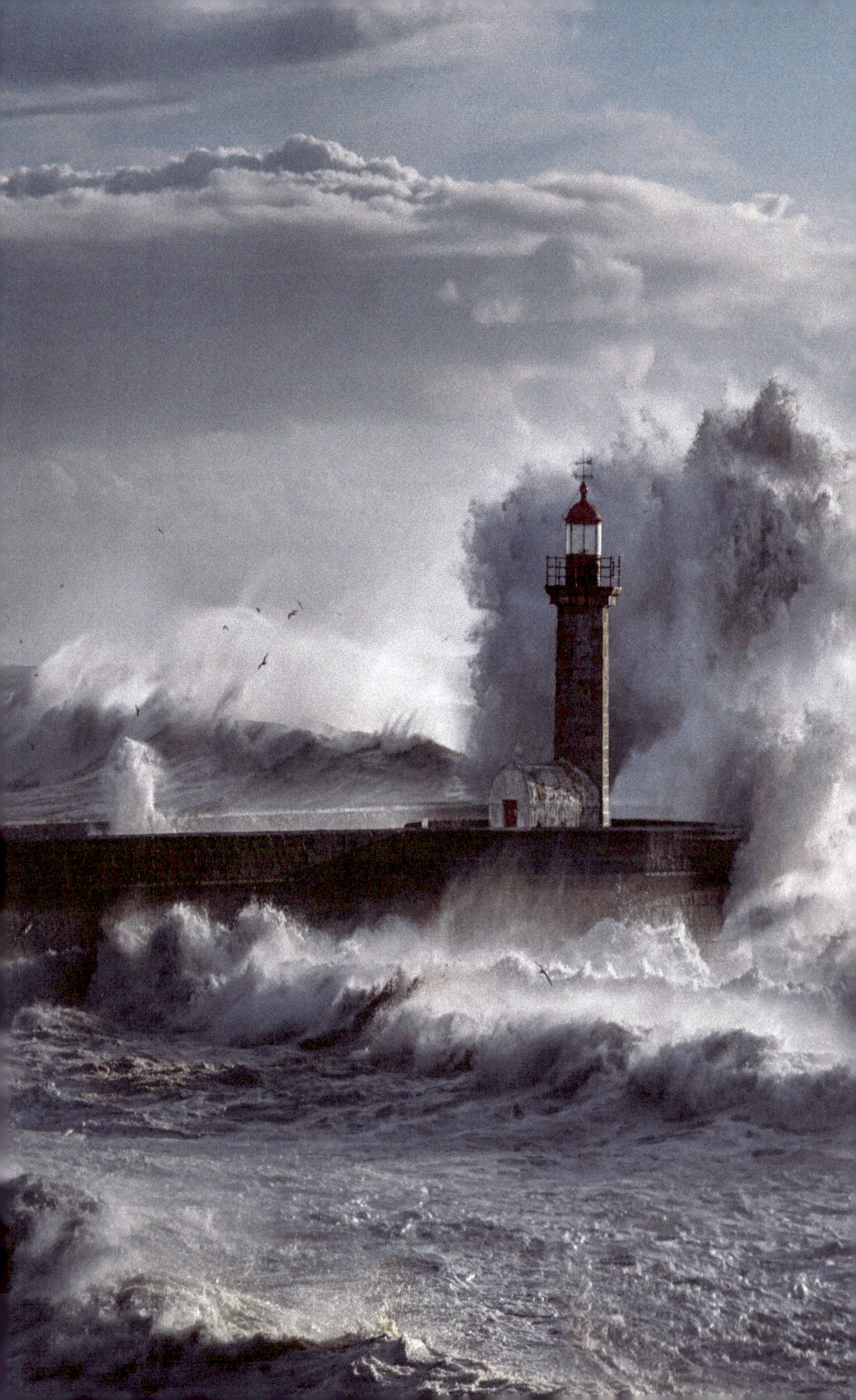

CHAPTER 21

When Challenges Overwhelm Facing the Hard Truths of Maturity

"You will always be the lighthouse."

Ease into the process gradually and with sensitivity

As individuals with Prader-Will Syndrome mature and their behavioural challenges evolve, it becomes crucial to adapt our strategies and adopt a more collaborative approach. Sensitivity and gradual implementation remain key factors in our success. Rather than imposing abrupt changes that may trigger behavioural issues, we opt for a measured approach, making slight adjustments to their routine while maintaining overall consistency. Alongside these subtle shifts, we introduce open-ended sentences, empowering them with choices and a sense of autonomy.

For example: "Did you want to go for a walk to the beach or park? Do you want to walk for 20 minutes, or if we walk for 45 minutes then we can get a healthy gelato ice cream?" We have implemented a slight change by going for a walk, and ideally, we advise them at least a day in advance so they know.

Notice how we give them a lower amount of time first, then we provide them with a higher more reasonable level of time and also a small healthy reward which you both can enjoy. Gelato is made with less fat and sugar and it is also churned at a slower speed than ice-cream so its lower in calorie count too. Doing daily walks is good for exercise and you can always finish off with a healthy drink, juice, or boost juice, or coconut water etc. Make it healthy, and it will work itself out.

For Aston-Martin we go on daily walks, and if I know I'm going to have problems with him not wanting to go, I offer choices, and one reward. So, for Monday afternoon, we go to Sandgate and we walk for 45 minutes to one hour along the beach, and at the end we have a small cup, one scoop of Gelato. He has already burnt calories and his metabolism rate is up.

The next day we do something similar, I take him to the Westfield shopping centre and we use the Kingpin, which is a games room. In there he enjoys the games which uses his hand, eye and brain coordination, and he needs to listen to instructions of the game — but he is having fun, and it's a great interactive and sensory session to have. These are small changes for Aston Martin's cognitive learning, as he needs to follow the game instructions and learn now the game itself operates, and we gradually ease these into our current daily routines.

Below are some approaches for "easing into" the strategies:

1. Introduce routines gradually, focusing on consistent wake-up and bedtime schedules first.
2. Meal plans should be introduced incrementally, starting with small, frequent meals and gradually incorporating healthy options and portion control.
3. Visual aids, such as schedules and timers, should be introduced slowly, beginning with simple and clear visual cues.
4. Behaviour management should start with positive reinforcement and small rewards, gradually introducing consistent consequences.

5. When dealing with aggressive behaviour, stay calm, maintain a non-threatening posture, and speak in a reassuring tone.
6. Ensure the environment is safe and offer the individual space and respect.
7. Redirect their attention to calming stimuli and provide verbal validation and empathy.
8. Encourage positive coping strategies and avoid physical restraint unless necessary for safety.
9. If issues persist, seek assistance from trained professionals and document incidents to develop proactive strategies.
10. Engage individuals in meaningful activities, allowing them to express preferences and find fulfillment.
11. Keep your communication sensitive, gentle and patient when conveying expectations and boundaries.
12. Involve professional support gradually to build comfort and trust.
13. Provide caregivers with respite and support services to maintain their wellbeing.
14. A gradual approach promotes trust, familiarity, and comfort with new routines, leading to a successful transition in managing behavioural challenges.

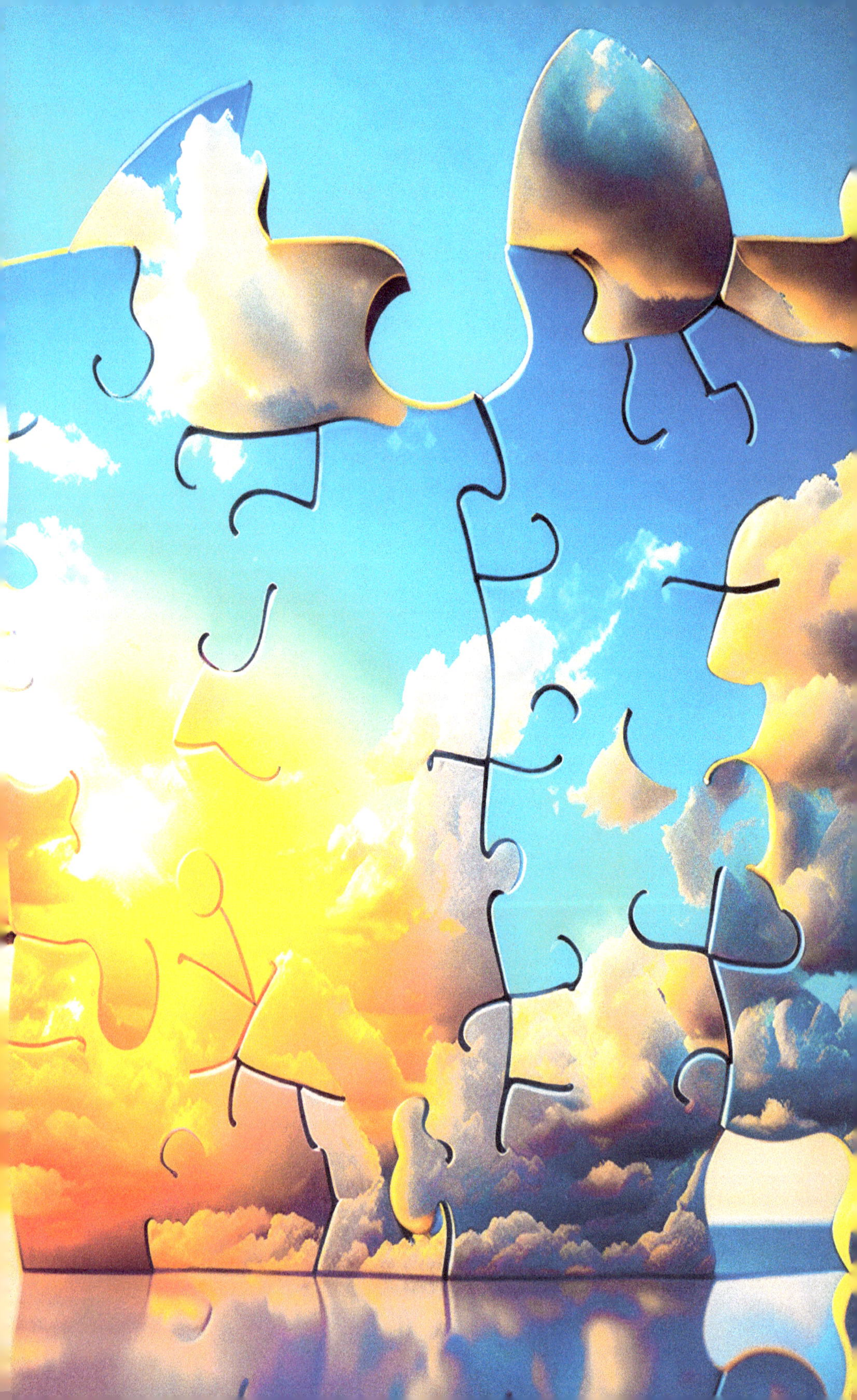

CHAPTER 22

Exploring Emotional Regulation with GABA and Concerta

In our quest to support Aston-Martin's wellbeing, we delved into the world of emotional regulation and the role of gamma-aminobutyric acid (GABA). Research suggested that individuals with Prader-Willi Syndrome may have lower GABA levels in their brains compared to typically developing individuals. This revelation sparked my intrigue, given the importance of GABA in modulating affective states and behavioural patterns.

The potential therapeutic benefits of GABA for individuals with PWS warranted further exploration. A critical review of a relevant research article enhanced our understanding: GABA, an amino acid, and neurotransmitter, plays a pivotal role in mediating neuronal communication and modulating brain activity, inducing a calming effect.

The hypothesis suggested that a deficiency in GABA could disrupt neurochemical signaling, leading to an imbalance in brain activity. We consulted Aston-Martin's pediatrician at the Queensland Children's Hospital, acknowledging the importance of individualized medical advice, especially with his unique condition of PWS with Subtype Uniparental Disomy (UPD).

The GABA Trial

We embarked on a 100-day trial of GABA supplementation for Aston-Martin, during which he took a daily GABA capsule. Our observations were meticulously documented, and his educator was kept informed to gather insights into any changes in his scholastic behaviour. The goal was to explore the potential synergistic effects of Concerta and GABA in modulating brain function, hoping for a therapeutic breakthrough.

The GABA supplement was sourced from a reputable company, Piping Rock Health Products, LLC®, approved by the Food and Drug Administration (FDA) in the United States. We opted for the 500mg, 100-tablet quick-release tablet formulation.

Understanding PWS Critical Region: The complexity of PWS lies in the 'critical region,' involving the GABA receptor subunit genes: GABRB3, GABRA5, and GABRG3. Individuals with PWS, including those with UPD, often show reduced paternal expression of GABRB3. This diminished expression impacts the development of GABAA receptors, with potential implications for brain function and behaviour.

Making the Connection: By understanding the six levels of disquietude in PWS children and their connection to GABA, I established a link between Aston-Martin's behavioural challenges and the potential benefits of GABA supplementation. The daily journal helped us to track his progress and adjust the dosage as needed.

One of the key goals was to improve Aston-Martin's emotional regulation by reasoning with him logically, helping him stay at a calm level without escalating his anxiety. However, his current struggle with logical reasoning, especially around food portions, presented a challenge. We observed that his desire for more food could quickly escalate from a calm state to higher levels of disquietude.

The Way Forward: The GABA trial, alongside the use of Concerta, holds promise for recalibrating Aston-Martin's therapeutic journey. While we remain optimistic, it is essential we closely monitor any changes and continue seeking guidance from medical professionals. Reading medical journals on PWS is highly recommended to deepen your understanding of the syndrome and its characteristics.

CHAPTER 22.1

A Hundred Days of Transformation: Aston-Martin's Journey with GABA

We decided to take a bold step and embark on a 100-day journey with Aston-Martin, introducing a combined approach of gamma-aminobutyric acid (GABA) supplementation and methylphenidate (Concerta) to address his behavioural challenges. GABA, being the major inhibitory neurotransmitter, holds the key to modulating neural excitability and signaling in the brain. With research suggesting a link between low GABA levels and temper outbursts, skin-picking, and autism-related behaviours in individuals with Prader-Willi Syndrome, we hoped for a positive impact.

The First Week: A subtle metamorphosis

As we began, Aston-Martin started his daily routine with GABA and Concerta. The initial signs of change were subtle yet noticeable. His educators reported a tranquil and cooperative demeanour at school, a deviation from his usual resistant responses. Over the first week, we observed a softening in his demeanour at home too, with increased serenity and composure. The combination of GABA and Concerta seemed to work synergistically, with GABA providing a calming influence that complemented Concerta's stimulatory effects.

As the days turned into weeks, a pattern emerged. Aston-Martin's mornings and evenings became notably calmer. He displayed a sunny disposition upon waking up, actively engaging in tasks like bed-making and breakfast preparation. The swiftness of GABA's effect brought a perceptible increment in his energy and playful mischief, a welcome change from his usual behavioural spectra.

The First Month: Managing upsets with ease

Over the first month, we witnessed a transformation in Aston-Martin's ability to manage upsets. While occasional outbursts occurred, they were less severe, rarely exceeding level 2 on the scale and occasionally reaching level 3. The duration of these upsets was shorter, giving me more time to intervene and de-escalate the situation. With the GABA supplement as the sole modification, I maintained our routine, and Aston-Martin's overall demeanour improved significantly.

The Sixth Week: Outbursts minimised, calmness prevails

By the sixth week, Aston-Martin's outbursts had become minimal, and his calmness prevailed. He found enjoyment in sensory play, and his absent seizures also showed a slight reduction. The initial dosage of 500mg GABA proved effective, and we had the option to increase it if needed. The positive changes brought a sense of gratification to both Aston-Martin and me.

The Eighth Week: Level-headed and resilient

As we entered the eighth week, Aston-Martin's mornings and evenings remained consistently calm. While there were occasional instances of upset, they rarely escalated beyond level 2 on the scale. The frequency of level 3 outbursts had reduced to about two per week, and de-escalating these situations became easier. I employed whispering, a calm demeanour, and gentle sensory touch to help him regulate his emotions effectively.

A calmer environment

Continuing into the following months, the positive impact of GABA was sustained. Aston-Martin's behaviour remained consistent, with calm mornings and evenings and only occasional upsets that were quickly resolved. The reduction in behavioural issues and the overall improvement in his demeanour were noticeable and rewarding. The changes observed brought hope and a commitment to continue monitoring his progress.

A journey towards emotional regulation

Over the 100 days, we witnessed a significant improvement in Aston-Martin's ability to manage and control his emotions. While not a panacea, the GABA supplement, in conjunction with Concerta, brought about a calmer and more enjoyable environment for both Aston-Martin and me. The changes were not absolute, but the slight improvements in his behavioural moods were a good start, and we plan to continue this treatment.

The journey towards emotional regulation is an ongoing process, and we remain hopeful that GABA will continue to play a positive role in Aston-Martin's development. The transformation observed thus far has been heartening, and we look forward to further progress and a brighter future for Aston-Martin.

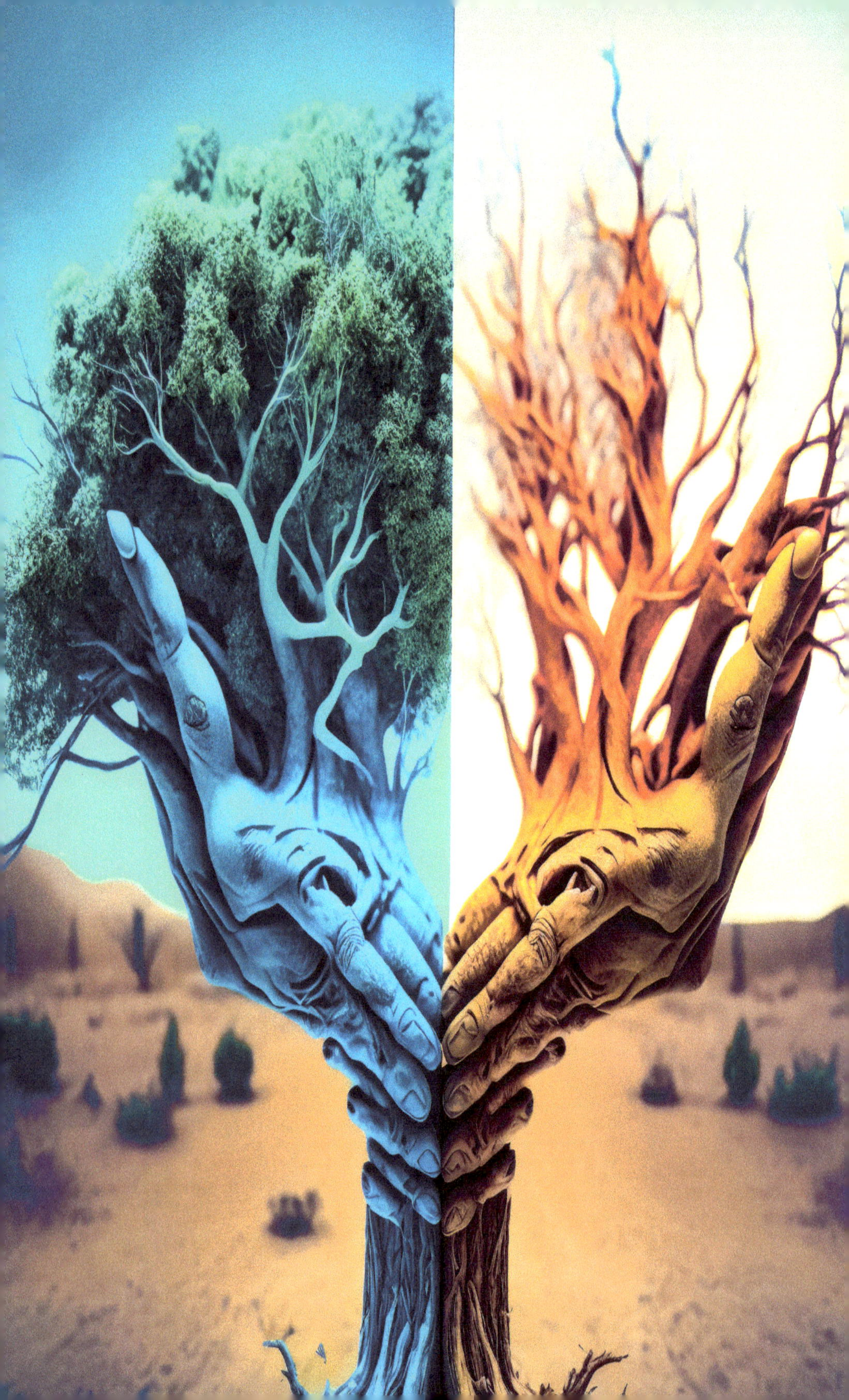

CHAPTER 23

Proposing an Advanced Diploma in Behavioural Therapy with a Genetic and Chromosomal Emphasis

In the progressive accumulation of years on our journey with Prader-Willi Syndrome, I have discerned a consequential gap in the preparatory training of magical guardians, the majority of whom have achieved their qualifications through the Certificate III or IV in Individual Disability Support. This division, most notably evident in their encounters with Prader-Willi Syndrome and related conditions, has prompted not just concern but an undeniable risk to the thoroughly customised care necessary for individuals such as Aston-Martin. This is through no fault of their own but due to the system requiring updates in the magical guardians' course work. I fully empathise for those magical guardians as they are true to the heart.

The designation "disability" envelopes a vast spectrum of divergent impairments, comprising physical, sensory, cognitive, or developmental forms that obstruct daily functional capacity and hinder societal participation. Varying in severity, these impairments may be congenital or acquired.

A recurrent predicament emerged as support professionals, despite a rudimentary exposition of PWS, displayed an observable pattern of either limited engagement with Aston-Martin or seeking refuge in outdoor spaces or other areas of the premises. The turnover of disability support workers who found themselves unequipped to contend with Aston-Martin's behavioural complexities became a telling trend. Some would resort to contacting me amid a behavioural crisis or noncompliance from Aston-Martin, necessitating my abrupt return to de-escalate the situation.

While the Certificate III and IV qualifications are commendable attempts to provide an introduction to the complex world of disability support, they may not sufficiently prepare support workers for the nuances associated with genetic and chromosomal aberrations. In the case of my son, Aston-Martin, it became evident that even the most dedicated and well-intentioned support workers, whom I fondly refer to as magical guardians, lacked the specialised knowledge and tools needed to manage his unique condition effectively.

The individual Disability support certificate programs offer a broad overview of the realm of complex genetic conditions and a diverse array of genetic syndromes. However, with over a thousand recognised syndromes, it is understandable that the curricula cannot delve into the intricacies of each one. As a result, graduates may receive a foundational understanding, along with advice to seek further insights from health professionals.

In Aston-Martin's situation, the limitations of these certificate programs became apparent. Despite the best efforts of the support workers, and God love them all, they found themselves unequipped to adequately address the complexities of his condition. This shortfall was not due to any fault of their own, but rather a reflection of the current curriculum's limitations. It created an unfortunate circumstance where both the support workers and my son were left without the specialised support they deserved.

I believe that enhancing the curriculum to include more specific training on rare genetic disorders, such as Prader-Will Syndrome, would better prepare future support workers. By recognising and addressing these gaps, we can ensure that individuals with rare genetic disorders receive the comprehensive support they need. It is important to acknowledge the dedication and compassion of the magical guardians (support workers) while also advocating for continuous improvement in the disability support sector.

The Advanced curriculum envisioned for this program aims to provide students with a deep understanding of genetic and chromosomal irregularities, shedding light on prevalent syndromes while also offering elective modules for exploring less common conditions. By doing so, we recognise the importance of equipping future support workers with a comprehensive knowledge base that prepares them for a wide range of scenarios they may encounter in their careers.

A unique aspect of this curriculum is the integration of sports therapy, which emphasises the roles of physical engagement in promoting holistic health. Within this framework, students will be trained to become sports coaches and exercise guides, utilising community parks as a setting for their practice. This approach not only promotes physical wellbeing but also creates a sense of community and inclusion for individuals with disabilities.

The pedagogical facet of the program mirrors the rigour and dedication exhibited by special schools' teacher's aides. Through immersive experiences, students will step into the lives of individuals across various disability categories, gaining first-hand understanding of their challenges and triumphs. This hands-on approach will foster the development of crucial skills in establishing structure, routine, and navigating complex learning processes, ensuring that graduates of the program are well-prepared to support individuals with disabilities effectively and compassionately.

Behavioural studies play a crucial role in this diploma program as they empower students with the skills to manage cognitive and behavioural challenges effectively. By incorporating these studies, students will gain insights into the mental schemas and decision-making processes of individuals with disabilities, fostering empathy and a deeper understanding of their needs. This knowledge will enable them to provide tailored support that aligns with various therapeutic disciplines, enhancing their credibility as therapy support professionals.

A qualification of this nature is ideal for individuals aspiring to become Educational Disability Sports Behavioural Therapists. These therapists will be equipped to work across diverse community contexts, including domiciliary and institutional settings. With this specialised training, they will become guardians of a sort, providing magic-like support that transforms lives.

By assuming the occupational mantle of Educational Disability Sports Behavioural Therapists, they will become agents of change, empowering their clients to overcome challenges and achieve their goals. The diploma program, with its focus on behavioural studies and holistic support, ensures that graduates are well-prepared to deliver magic-like transformations in the lives of those they support.

Expanding the new circle of influence

Over time and with gathered expertise, the new cadre of disability support workers will accrue an expansive understanding of both the aetiology of complex syndromes and the most effective management strategies.

While adherence to routine remains pivotal for PWS individuals' care, a deeper exploration into these complex conditions is imperative for discerning and managing the attendant behavioural intricacies. It stands to reason that cases with intricate genetic and chromosomal blueprints would profoundly benefit from the expertise of a therapist with indispensable tailored education and steeped in the nuances of genetically-derived variations.

I imagine that the course proposed concept would be subject to a comprehensive evaluation by the Australian Skills Quality Authority (ASQA). Such scrutiny would solidify the integrity of curricular content, pedagogical design, stakeholders, research and the underlying theoretical principles. After meticulous review and validation, I hope that this curricular framework will permeate the discipline of disability support through Registered Training Organisations (RTOs) and Technical and Further Education (TAFE) institutes across the nation.

For those interested, further details of my proposed course concepts are outlined in Appendix A.

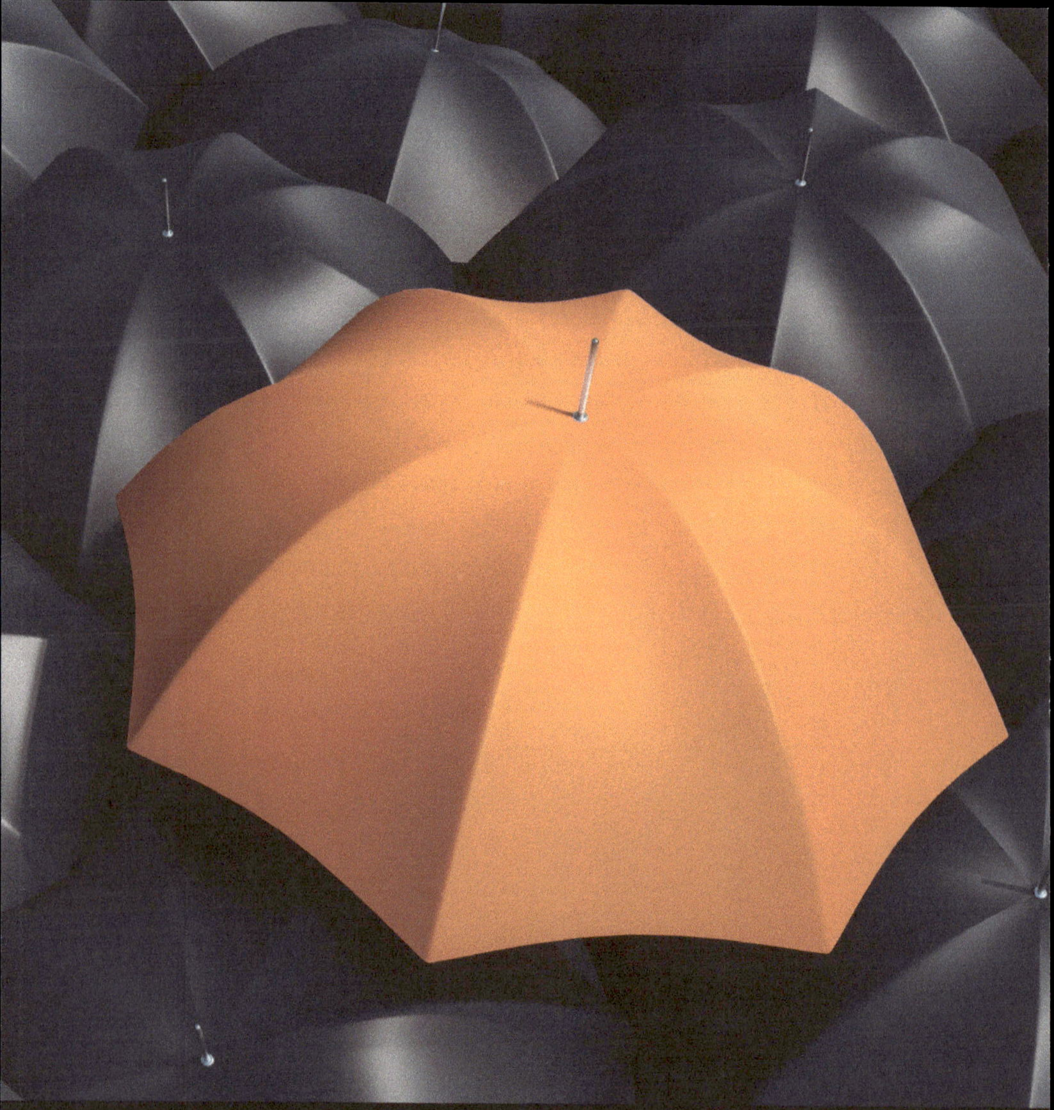

One in eight billion

CHAPTER 24

You're my one in 8 billion - My closing moments

It's like someone picked you out of the sky, there is always a reason why events happen. Supporting a person with Prader-Willi Syndrome is a unique and special journey filled with love, patience and joy. It's as if they were chosen for a wonderful and beautiful life, and as their caregiver, you have been selected to bring out the best in them. While raising a child with PWS presents its challenges, it has also been an amazing, fun and rewarding experience. The past decade has been a testament to the best of my capabilities, and I would choose this path again without hesitation. For Aston-Martin: you're my one in 8 billion.

When caring for a child with PWS, you need to understand their unique needs and provide them with the time and patience they require. Structure and routine are paramount, if you don't have these in place, then your job becomes harder. Not everything is always going to work, and you need to experiment and find answers as to what works and what does not.

It can be challenging to manage their feelings of frustration and disappointment, but I found that creating a positive, supportive environment is key. Using positive language and expressing genuine interest in their desires can help create a calming atmosphere. Additionally, speaking to your PWS child in a calm, understanding manner and showing empathy can aid in their quick recovery from distressing situations.

Aston-Martin, for example, often seeks fairness and can become upset when faced with perceived injustices. By acknowledging his feelings and expressing understanding, I can help him navigate these emotions and maintain a sense of calm. Avoiding direct and confrontational language, and instead offering choices and opportunities for control, has proven to be more effective in managing his behaviour and promoting a positive environment.

It's important to remember that each individual with PWS may respond differently, and it's essential to approach each situation with patience, love and understanding. By creating a supportive and positive environment, we can help individuals with PWS thrive and lead fulfilling lives.

In managing one of the more prevalent challenges, hyperphagia, I found that by establishing clear meal and snack times, Aston-Martin felt more secure in knowing nourishment will be provided regularly. Being flexible can be difficult, so I found sticking to schedules was beneficial. Eating every few hours allows Aston-Martin's calorie needs to be met in a balanced way.

With open communication, compassion and teamwork, we can create an environment that supports wellness, independence and happiness for individuals with PWS each and every day. Their quality of life depends on consistency from their community of caregivers.

I think we are all chosen to accomplish something special in life, and the birth of your child signifies that you have the perfect traits to bring this child into the world and deliver the best of them. To me, it's like they were pre-chosen, giving them a chance at a wonderful and beautiful life. Bringing up a child is never easy, a child with PWS is going to be even more challenging. For me, the last 10 years have been a challenging, amazing, fun, joyful, upsetting, emotional ride.

If I could give some final takeaways from this, it would be that when you look after a child with PWS, they are unique, but you need to give yourself time to develop an understanding of how they work.

Framing responses with an optimistic, future-oriented tone demonstrates care and understanding for their perspective. Solutions that acknowledge feelings and offer a balanced compromise model healthy emotion regulation. With compassion, and by making their emotional wellbeing a top priority, caregivers can effectively support those living with PWS in navigating everyday frustrations.

I found that I needed to develop overall **strategies**, such as taking Aston-Martin for a walk to the park every day for social interaction and social cues teachings, but also **tactics** to deploy in a hurry as a deflection, such as bringing out the colouring books and helping him use the correct colours for the picture's environments, so the sky is blue and not green, or teaching him to colour in between the lines and learning how to write his name through tracing letters and numbers. Other tactics I used include playing games in the back yard or catching 'ants' which he likes, or butterflies, and examining those in a container with the intention to release them back into the wild. Small tactics in the home will help them learn social cues. As I mentioned previously, 'pick your battles' — which means using tactics to sometimes rescue your overall strategies.

Medication is worth investigating, as if it is effective, this will help them and you. I use Concerta 54mg and GABA supplement tablets daily to help Aston-Martin to keep calm, and to focus. This does work, but its more trial and error with the GABA to find the right dosage, and its best to speak with your doctor about this one.

Over the preceding decade, my intellectual and emotional faculties have undergone a rigorous tutorial in the intricacies of Prader-Willi Syndrome — a term that muscled its way into my lexicon with the subtlety of a linguistic bulldozer at precisely 22:26 on the 15th of August 2013. Before this momentous timestamp, the condition was as alien to me as a hypothetical fourteenth month in the annual calendar.

The saga with Aston-Martin, much like grappling with a Rubik's cube in the dark, has prodded my awareness to Herculean levels and imparted erudition in a domain I once presumed beyond my intellectual grasp. The quest, spanning a decade, has seen me voraciously devouring medical tomes and journals in pursuit of enlightenment and, audaciously, a panacea that tantalisingly whispers the name 'Gene therapy'.

Navigating this odyssey, primarily to decrypt my son's cosmos from the parental gaze, has been a labour akin to translating a novel without a cipher. The arduous undertaking of marshalling a cadre of individuals adept at reinforcing our battlements in this undertaking has presented a challenge of Herculean proportions; after all, not every soul is cut out for the tapestry of a PWS child's unique universe.

Possessed of a steely resolve, I have immersed myself in the annals of medical literature, enhancing my comprehension of his condition and thus fortifying my arsenal to escort Aston-Martin toward his milestones. The buck, as they say, stops with me — every decision I make for his wellbeing, his requirements, and the recalibration of his life trajectory to a frequency he can decode, rests weightily upon my shoulders. Indeed, life within this complex PWS labyrinth is not for the faint of heart.

This is not the tale of an acquired neurocognitive shift at a decade's milestone, replete with pre-injury memories serving as breadcrumbs back to former selves. Rather, for Aston-Martin, the reality he was born into is his baseline — the only template of existence he knows.

To bridge the interstellar gap in understanding, we, his navigators and guardians, must immerse ourselves in his cosmos, decoding his thought processes before charting and embarking on a course of action. Such is the life less ordinary, one not of seamless, smooth sailing, but rather, a voyage through richer, more formidable seas of knowledge.

It is my earnest aspiration that perusing the pages of this tome has augmented your understanding and knowledge of Prader-Willi Syndrome and that it has, in some capacity, served as a beacon in the oftentimes murky waters of comprehension.

I thank you from my heart for going through this journey with me.

Those with PWS or any other syndrome, are all special people in their own unique way. I took the time to write a song and have them turned into a song — for Aston-Martin and also for all special needs people within the community where ever you maybe.

The song is on *Spotify, Apple Music, iTunes, Instagram/Facebook, TikTok & other ByteDance stores, YouTube Music, Amazon, Pandora, Deezer, Tidal, iHeartRadio, Claro Música, Saavn, Boomplay, Anghami, NetEase, Tencent, Qobuz, Joox, Kuack Media, Adaptr, Flo, MediaNet, Snapchat* and is titled: **'One in 8Billion'**.

The song is sung by a Fiverr's UK female artist named Christina **@christinartnd**. She is a professional Female Singer and vocalist in the United Kingdom.

The song is produced by Fiverr's Marvin **@mfmusicprod** a professional Dutch producer, songwriter, guitarist and vocalist. I would like to thank them for an absolutely amazing job they both did; teamwork makes the dream work. I encourage you to listen to and enjoy the song.

Sebastiaan Van Nuissenburg

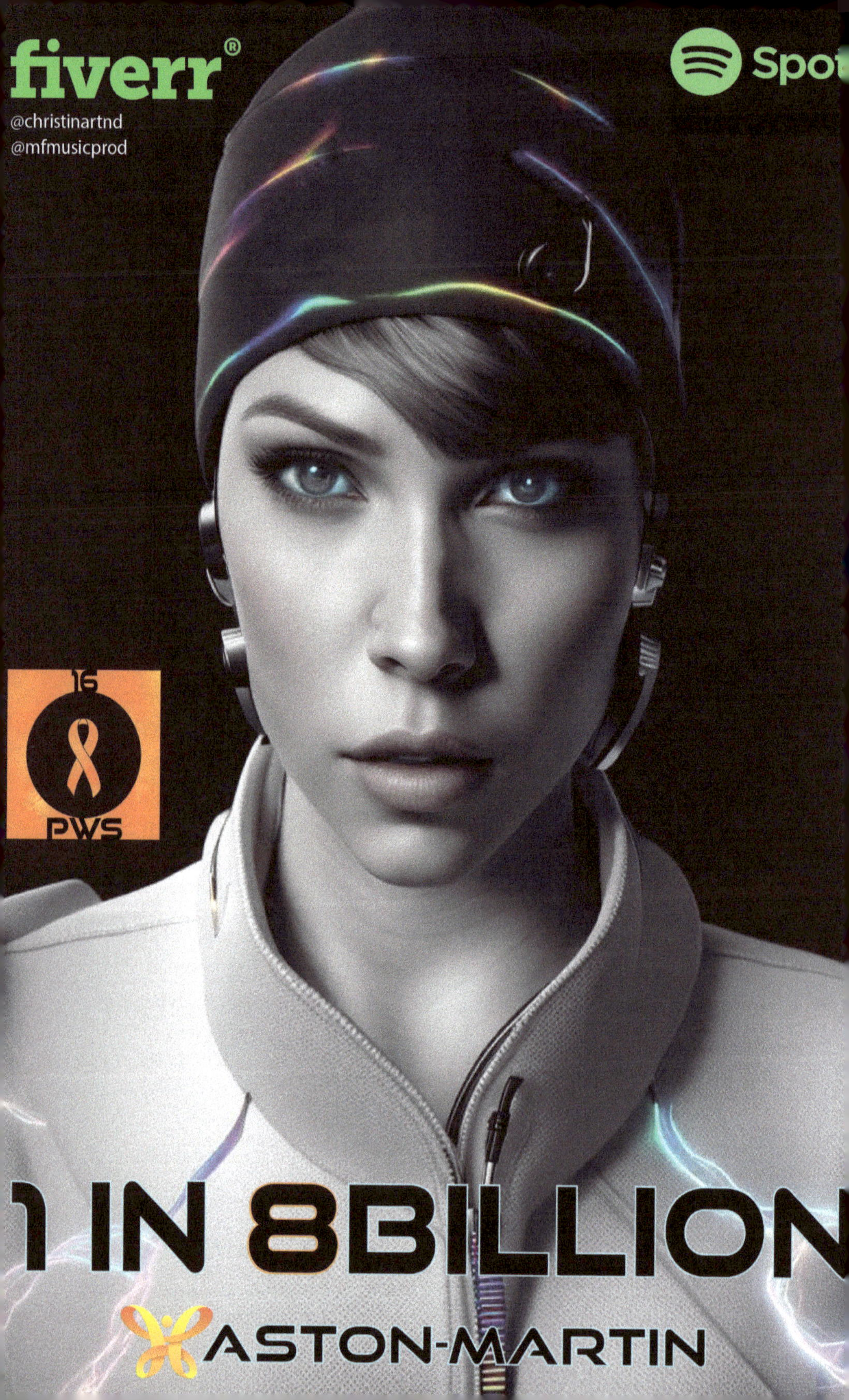
fiverr®
@christinartnd
@mfmusicprod
Spot
16
PWS
1 IN 8BILLION
ASTON-MARTIN

Bibliography

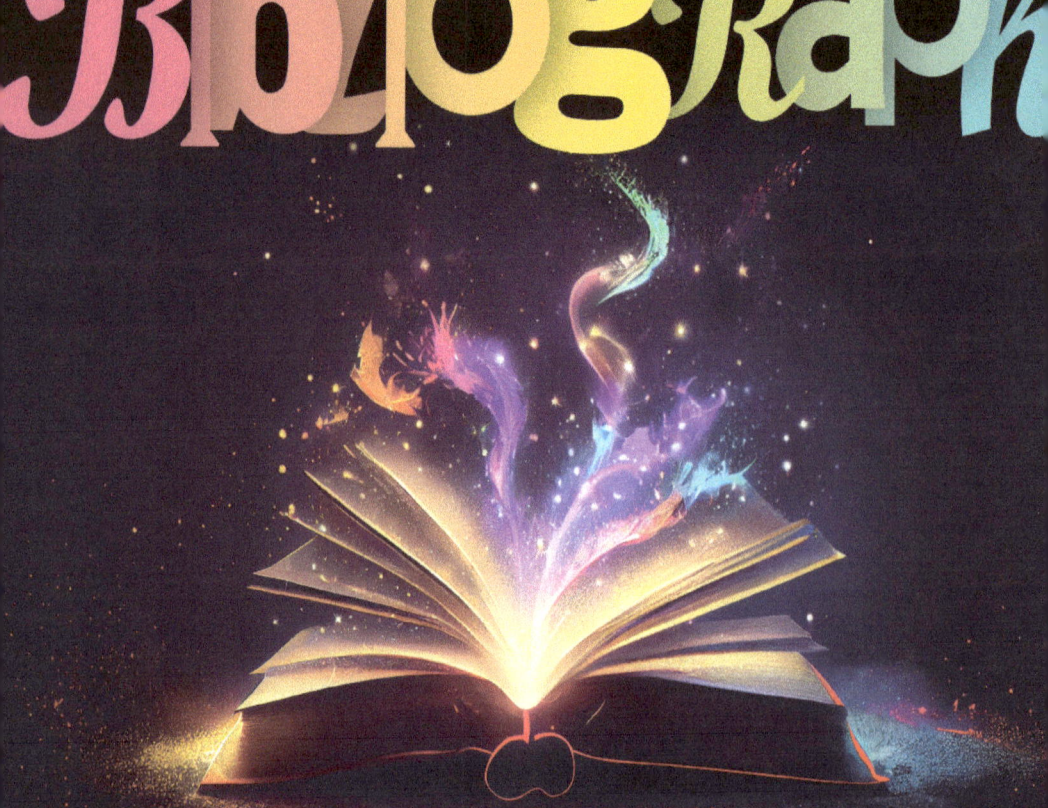

Bibliography

1) "Angelman Syndrome." *Vic.gov.au*, 2012, www.betterhealth.vic.gov.au/health/conditionsandtreatments/angelman-syndrome.

2) Angulo, M. A., et al. "Prader-Willi Syndrome: A Review of Clinical, Genetic, and Endocrine Findings." *Journal of Endocrinological Investigation*, vol. 38, no. 12, 11 June 2015, pp. 1249–1263, dx.doi.org/10.1007%2Fs40618-015-0312-9, https://doi.org/10.1007/s40618-015-0312-9. Accessed 21 Nov. 2019.

3) Australian Bureau of Statistics. (2020, September 25). Disability, Ageing and Carers, Australia: Summary of Findings, 2018 | Australian Bureau of Statistics. www.abs.gov.au. https://www.abs.gov.au/statistics/health/disability/disability-ageing-and-carers-australia-summary-findings/latest-release#disabilityButler, Merlin G., et al. "Prader-Willi Syndrome - Clinical Genetics, Diagnosis and Treatment Approaches: An Update." *Current Pediatric Reviews*, vol. 15, 16 July 2019, https://doi.org/10.2174/1573396315666190716120925.

4) ——. "Prader-Willi Syndrome - Clinical Genetics, Diagnosis and Treatment Approaches: An Update." *Current Pediatric Reviews*, vol. 15, 16 July 2019, https://doi.org/10.2174/1573396315666190716120925.

5) Buttermore, Elizabeth D, et al. "16p13.11 Deletion Variants Associated with Neuropsychiatric Disorders Cause Morphological and Synaptic Changes in Induced Pluripotent Stem Cell-Derived Neurons." *Frontiers in Psychiatry*, vol. 13, 3 Nov. 2022, https://doi.org/10.3389/fpsyt.2022.924956. Accessed 17 Sept. 2023.

6) Cai, Meiying, et al. "16p13.11 Microdeletion/Microduplication in Fetuses: Investigation of Associated Ultrasound Phenotypes, Genetic Anomalies, and Pregnancy Outcome Follow-Up." *BMC Pregnancy and Childbirth*, vol. 22, no. 1, 7 Dec. 2022, www.ncbi.nlm.nih.gov/

pmc/articles/PMC9727942/, https://doi.org/10.1186/s12884-022-05267-w. Accessed 15 Nov. 2023.

7) Fujitani, M, et al. "A Chromosome 16p13.11 Microduplication Causes Hyperactivity through Dysregulation of MiR-484/Protocadherin-19 Signaling." *Molecular Psychiatry*, vol. 22, no. 3, 5 July 2016, pp. 364–374, https://doi.org/10.1038/mp.2016.106. Accessed 1 Dec. 2020.

8) Grootjen, Lionne N., et al. "Prenatal and Neonatal Characteristics of Children with Prader-Willi Syndrome." *Journal of Clinical Medicine*, vol. 11, no. 3, 28 Jan. 2022, p. 679, mdpi-res.com/d_attachment/jcm/jcm-11-00679/article_deploy/jcm-11-00679.pdf?version=1643357227, https://doi.org/10.3390/jcm11030679.

9) Heinzen, Erin L., et al. "Rare Deletions at 16p13.11 Predispose to a Diverse Spectrum of Sporadic Epilepsy Syndromes." *American Journal of Human Genetics*, vol. 86, no. 5, 14 May 2010, pp. 707–718, pubmed.ncbi.nlm.nih.gov/20398883/, https://doi.org/10.1016/j.ajhg.2010.03.018. Accessed 3 May 2023.

10) Liu, Shu, et al. "Uniparental Disomy of Chromosome 15 in Two Cases by Chromosome Microarray: A Lesson Worth Thinking." *Cytogenetic and Genome Research*, vol. 152, no. 1, 2017, pp. 1–8, https://doi.org/10.1159/000477520. Accessed 12 Feb. 2022.

11) Mageau, Geneviève A, and Robert J Vallerand. "The Coach–Athlete Relationship: A Motivational Model." *Journal of Sports Sciences*, vol. 21, no. 11, Nov. 2003, pp. 883–904, selfdeterminationtheory.org/wp-content/uploads/2014/04/2003_MageauVallerand_Coach.pdf, https://doi.org/10.1080/0264041031000140374.

12) "Media Release - Australia's Birth Rate Falls, but Older Mothers Buck the Trend (Media Release)." *Abs.gov.au*, c=AU; o=Commonwealth of Australia; ou=Australian Bureau of Statistics, 2013, www.abs.gov.au/ausstats/abs@.nsf/lookup/3301.0Media%20Release12013. Accessed 17 Nov. 2023.

13) Schwartz, Lauren, et al. "Behavioural Features in Prader-Willi Syndrome (PWS): Consensus Paper from the International PWS Clinical Trial Consortium." *Journal of Neurodevelopmental Disorders*, vol. 13, no. 1, 21 June 2021, p. 25, pubmed.ncbi.nlm.nih.gov/34148559/#:~:text=Prader%2DWilli%20syndrome%20(PWS), https://doi.org/10.1186/s11689-021-09373-2.

14) Smith, Amanda Elizabeth, et al. "Chromosome 16p13.11 Microdeletion Syndrome in a Newborn: A Case Study." *Neonatal Network*, vol. 37, no. 5, Sept. 2018, pp. 303–309, https://doi.org/10.1891/0730-0832.37.5.303. Accessed 26 May 2021.
15) "Unique | Understanding Rare Chromosome and Gene Disorders." *Unique*, rarechromo.org/.
16) Zhang, Lu, et al. "Genetic Subtypes and Phenotypic Characteristics of 110 Patients with Prader-Willi Syndrome." *Italian Journal of Pediatrics*, vol. 48, no. 1, 23 July 2022, https://doi.org/10.1186/s13052-022-01319-1. Accessed 15 Nov. 2022.

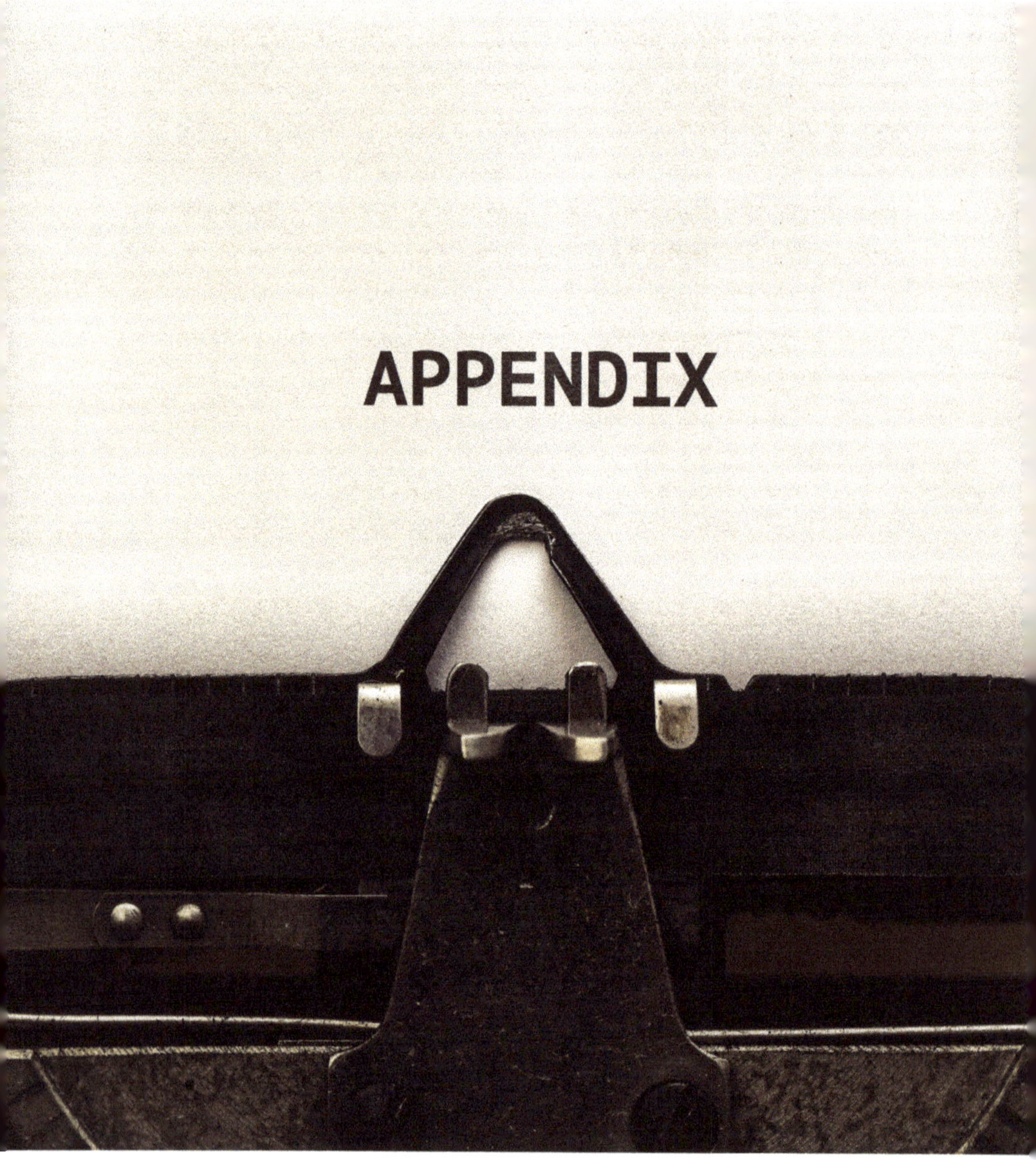
APPENDIX

Appendix A

Appendix A: Linked to Chapter 23, proposing an Advanced Diploma in Behavioural Therapy with a Genetic and Chromosomal Emphasis.

Graduates of this program will emerge as pioneers, armed with a comprehensive toolkit that includes incisive understanding, advanced skills, and a client-centric approach. They will be prepared to navigate the intricacies of rare genetic disorders and provide tailored support that fosters independence and maximises potential. The proposed course bridges the gap between academic knowledge and real-world application, ensuring graduates are well-versed in evidence-based practices that drive positive change and will continuously evolve to enhance the wellbeing of their clients.

One of the key strengths of this advanced diploma is its focus on bridging academia and clinical expertise. By bringing together theoretical foundations and practical, evidence-based strategies, graduates will become vanguards of holistic, personalised care. They will not only improve outcomes for individuals with rare genetic disorders but also contribute to community inclusivity and promote a paradigm shift towards more effective and satisfying support services.

Through cross-sector collaboration, this advanced diploma has the potential to revolutionise the NDIS landscape in Australia. It will equip therapists, educators, and support workers with specialised training, enhancing the multi-disciplinary approach and directly benefiting Australian families affected by rare genetic disorders.

By embracing this innovative curriculum, we take a giant step forward in addressing the complex needs of individuals with chromosomal and genetic abnormalities. The advanced Diploma in Behavioral Therapy for Rare Genetic Disorders is designed to produce highly skilled professionals who are passionate about making a meaningful impact, ensuring that individuals with rare genetic disorders receive the dedicated support they deserve.

Course unit summary

12 units must be completed:
9 core units
3 elective units

Course insights

Estimated duration 18 month(s) - 2 year(s)

Core Units (9)

Here are 9 core units with brief outlines for the Advanced Diploma in Behavioural Therapy as an Educational and Disability Sports Therapist for Rare Genetic Disorders:

Module one: Provide individual educational assistance in a structured environment with Introduction to Intellectual Disability

Module Two: Foundations of Augmentative and Alternative Communication

Module three: Introduction to Behaviour Management

Module Four: Introduction to Individual Sports/Nutrition Coaching

Module Five: Facilitate Brain and Behavioural Management

Module Six: Anatomy and Physiology understanding

Module Seven: Cytogenetic, Genetics, Chromosome Abnormalities/conditions with intellectual disability

Module Eight: Treatment and Management of Genetic, Chromosome Abnormalities

Module nine: Management of life with a syndrome.

Electives: (3)

1. Supporting Individuals with Trisomy Syndromes
2. Supporting Individuals with Down Syndrome (Trisomy 21)
3. Supporting Individuals with Turner Syndrome
4. Supporting Individuals with Klinefelter Syndrome
5. Supporting Individuals with Fragile X Syndrome
6. Supporting Individuals with Marfan Syndrome
7. Supporting Individuals with Noonan Syndrome
8. Supporting Individuals with Williams Syndrome
9. Supporting Individuals with Prader-Willi Syndrome/ Angelman Syndrome
10. Supporting Individuals with Rett Syndrome
11. Supporting Individuals with Cri du Chat Syndrome
12. Supporting Individuals with Kleefstra Syndrome
13. Supporting Individuals with Neurofibromatosis

Some examples of what students would learn in the different modules could be:

1. **Introduction to Medical Genetics and Genomics** Outline: Overview of genetics concepts, genomic testing methods, inheritance patterns, genetic variation and risk assessment.
2. **Principles of Behavioural Therapy for Genetic Disorders** Outline: Principles of applied behaviour analysis, developmental approaches, functional behaviour assessment and positive behaviour support strategies.

3. **Nutritional and Dietary Management of Genetic Disorders** Outline: Role of nutrition in symptom management, specialised formula and supplement needs, feeding difficulties and relationship to behaviours.
4. **Communication Strategies across Genetic Disorders** Outline: Augmentative aids, alternative and assistive communication methods, addressing auditory processing issues and specific syndrome profiles.
5. **Physical and Occupational Therapy Approaches** Outline: Adapted physical activities, motor planning strategies, sensory integration techniques, orthopaedic and medical needs.
6. **Environmental Design and Management Strategies** Outline: Sensory considerations, routines and structure, safety modifications, transition supports and reducing behavioural triggers.
7. **Counselling and Family Systems Support** Outline: Sibling impacts, self-care strategies, grief and acceptance models, advocacy skills and community networking.
8. **Case Management and Crisis Prevention Planning** Outline: Multidisciplinary teams, compiling client histories and emergency protocols, goal setting and transition planning.
9. **Ethical and Professional Practice Standards** Outline: Responsibilities and competencies, cultural awareness, consent, disclosure and confidentiality.
10. **Research Literacy and Evidence-Based practice** Outline: Critically appraising research, finding and assessing evidence, principles of research ethics.

Some sample elective units and brief outlines are below:

1. **Management of Angelman Syndrome** Outline: Overview of genetic cause, phenotype in Angelman syndrome, behavioural implications and proven therapy approaches.
2. **Behavioural Issues in Cri du Chat Syndrome** Outline: Genetic deletion, common challenges, addressing self-injurious and aggression behaviours through environmental adaptations.
3. **Prader-Willi Syndrome:** A Multisystem Approach Outline: Genetic underpinnings, involvement of multiple medical specialists, therapies targeting physical, cognitive and behavioural features.
4. **Neurofibromatosis:** A Clinical Perspective Outline: Genotype-phenotype correlations in NF1 and NF2, adjustments to risk factors, symptom surveillance and allied health needs.
5. **Supporting Individuals with Kleefstra Syndrome** Outline: Rare deletion syndrome, presentations at different developmental levels, specialised educational programming and skill development strategies.

In conclusion, the proposed Advanced Diploma in Behavioral Therapy as an Educational and Disability Sports Therapists for Rare Genetic Disorders represents a transformative leap forward in addressing the complex educational and therapeutic needs of individuals with chromosomal and genetic abnormalities. This course goes beyond the foundations laid by Certificates III and IV in individual Disability Support by integrating specialised knowledge with empathetic and effective application strategies.

The curriculum has been meticulously designed to equip students with a nuanced understanding of rare genetic disorders and the skills to address their unique challenges. By delving into medical genetics, nutritional management, communication, and behavioural therapy specific to various syndromes, this advanced diploma empowers students to become rigorous professionals capable of making a profound difference.

www.ingramcontent.com/pod-product-compliance
Lightning Source LLC
Chambersburg PA
CBHW041137110526
44590CB00027B/4049